LIFE IS SHORT
LAUNDRY
IS ETERNAL

Confessions of a Stay-at-Home Dad

BY SCOTT BENNER

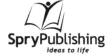

SpryPublishing
ideas to life

This edition is published by Spry Publishing LLC
2500 South State Street
Ann Arbor, MI 48104 USA

Printed and bound in the United States.

Library of Congress Control Number: 2012955674

10 9 8 7 6 5 4 3 2 1

Paperback ISBN: 978-1-938170-15-7
E-book ISBN: 978-1-938170-16-4

For and because of Kelly, Cole, and Arden

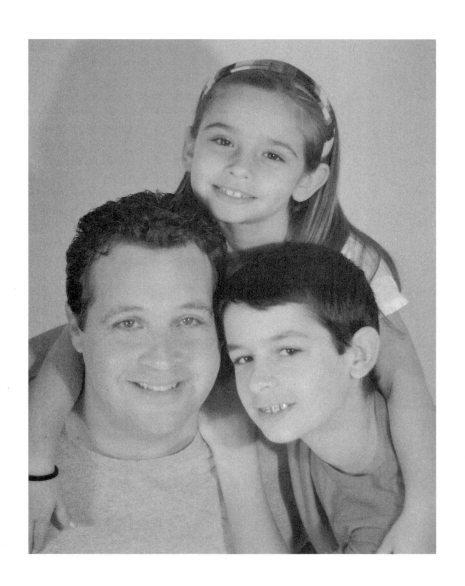

Author's Note

Life Is Short, Laundry Is Eternal was born out of my genuine desire to introduce both men and women to the world on the opposite side of the parental gender gap. We all live our lives so close to each other every day, but our perspectives and the preconceptions that we judge with ever skew our view of the other's world.

Rife with misconceptions, the life of a stay-at-home parent is often mocked but very rarely appreciated by the people who benefit most from that parent's dedicated work and persistence. Far too many think of this noblest of professions as easy, women's work, or, at best, secondary to the task of making a living. Being a stay-at-home parent is by far the most rewarding experience of my life, and I want you to see it through my eyes. Our children's growth is a marvel to behold, and shepherding them to the moment when we as parents hand them off to life is a transformational journey that I wish for every adult. From my son Cole's conception to the diagnosis of my daughter Arden's type 1 diabetes, I couldn't help but to give my heart over to the family that my wife Kelly and I created.

Life Is Short, Laundry Is Eternal is my unfiltered account of the moments that shape a family. There is simply no better career in the world than being a stay-at-home parent. If you don't believe me now, you will when you've finished reading my confessions.

Contents

Laundry Is Indeed Eternal

I think that I know why people become nudists—to have less laundry. Some quick math tells me that I complete an average of fifteen loads of laundry a week or more than sixty a month. That's more than seven hundred a year and nearly nine thousand in my time as a stay-at-home dad. In fact, by the time this book is published I'll have washed, dried, folded, and put away another almost thousand loads of laundry, and each one sucks a little more than the last.

Doing the laundry is so terrible that if a genie popped out of a bottle right now and said to me, "Answer fast, no more laundry or world peace—choose!" I'd actually pause before I responded, "World peace." And,

I guarantee that there would be days in the future while I was living in our new utopian and peaceful world that I'd regret my decision. That moment would likely come after a particularly long session of sort, fold, and put away.

In the laundry, shirts are evidence of your eating mistakes and rub up into your armpits. Pants are heavy, and they often take longer to dry than the rest of the load. Socks smell like, well, socks, and grabbing a sweaty one that hasn't completely dried when you are loading the machine makes you reconsider every life choice that brought you to that moment. That's right—a cold, damp sock has caused me to reconsider more than once my life's path.

And then there's underwear ... In what other walk of life would you consider removing your underwear, tossing them (hopefully) into a basket, and then assuming that someone will refresh them for you without compensation? No other. As an adult you wouldn't ask your mother, brother, priest, boss, or the guy who changes your oil to handle this task, but for some reason we don't think twice about asking our spouses to do it. Think back to when you were dating the person whom you're married to today.

Did you ever let that person see your dirty clothes? Would you have left a smelly shirt on the bed? I bet not. However, a few "I dos" later, and you are tossing your clothes around like there is a magic elf to bring them back clean.

Some of you miss the laundry basket and don't rebound. Others like to leave clothes on the floor next to the bed or in the living room. I had to purchase a large wicker basket for our family room so that my family could have a place to put their shoes. I, of course, thought that the bedroom closet that was provided would be a great place to put those shoes, but things never worked out quite that way. At least now when they abandon them in favor of another pair, it's easier for me to carry them upstairs and put them away.

Doing the laundry is the worst domestic task that I have ever encountered, but it's also a wonderful window into how working and stay-at-home spouses unfairly judge one another.

Recently my son Cole played a baseball game on a dreary Saturday afternoon. There was a huge storm system headed our way, but the rain held off long enough for the boys to play. With the storm bearing down there was little chance that they'd be able to get their next game in on the following day, so I didn't rush to do the laundry after Saturday's game.

Of course it never did rain that night, at least not hard enough to cancel the game on Sunday.

How did my son Cole show up with a clean uniform? The previous night around 1:30 AM when I was quietly checking Arden's blood glucose level and making an adjustment to her insulin, I noticed that I didn't hear the rain outside as I had expected. It was in that silence that I realized that I had never washed Cole's baseball uniform. So I put in a load of laundry, knowing that I'd be up for at least an hour to watch over Arden's blood glucose level. When the wash cycle finished, I moved the load to the dryer, checked on Arden once more, and finally went back to sleep.

When the topic of clean uniforms came up at Sunday's game and I recounted my story, one of the fathers turned to a mother and said, "See, he does the laundry in the middle of the night and doesn't complain about it." He clearly didn't think that doing the laundry was in anyway a tough task.

Before the mother could respond, I stepped back into the conversation and tried to explain why doing the laundry is so terrible. It seems that the spouse who goes to work outside of the house doesn't think that doing the laundry is any big deal. It's even considered a joke, especially in comparison to the tasks and pressures that the other spouse faces. In the end, hearing from another man how unpleasant, time consuming, and soul-sucking the task really is didn't help sway the man one bit.

In my life I've worked in retail, done landscaping, and was a baker. I even operated an industrial steel saw when I was in my early twenties. In the few years that I ran that saw, I almost cut off the pointer finger on my right hand. I burned a hole in the top of my foot, went blind for a weekend from welder's flash, and sliced a gash in my left palm that required hundreds of stitches. Please listen to me when I say this ... doing the laundry repeatedly for countless years is worse than all of that combined! I am not exaggerating, gilding the lily, or even telling a tale out of school. Plainly, sorting the laundry, folding the laundry, and putting away the laundry is the scourge of my existence.

When our home was redesigned, I only asked for one improvement. It wasn't a media room or a man cave. I asked if it was possible to put the laundry room on the second floor. I even had the builder pack its walls with soundproofing insulation so I could use the machines while my family slept. The architect remarked at the time that I was the only man who ever showed an interest in where the laundry room would be. I asked him how many of the men he met were stay-at-home dads, and he couldn't think of one.

I thought the same thing that day that I do now. Women aren't interested in where the laundry room is because they are women; they are interested because they are the ones who generally get stuck doing the laundry. I care about not having to walk up and down a thousand steps a week with a giant basket of clothes in my arms, but in the end I don't care about the laundry. I'm just the guy who does it.

Tomorrow when you're getting dressed, hold your drawers in the air and thank the person who washed them for you. It will really brighten her (or his) day, and not just because you'll look ridiculous standing naked holding your underwear over your head, for there is no more thankless task than making another's clothes clean again.

What Is a Family?

Over the course of my life and particularly during the twelve years I've been a stay-at-home dad, I've had a lot of time to ponder that question. To me, family means a group of people who love and protect each other. Structurally, I don't see any limitations on what a family is or can be. A mom and a dad, two moms, a single dad, being raised by your grandparents ... a family is a family.

My understanding of family began in July of 1971. I was born that month to a young girl who didn't believe she could give me the life that I deserved. For the next month until a family could be found to adopt me, a kind lady with good handwriting took care of me. I know she had good handwriting because she left a note for my eventual parents that began, "Here are just a few things about the baby to make your first days together a little easier ..." The lady with the nice handwriting went on to say that I got a little fussy in between meals; I liked bathing; and, not surprising to anyone who knows me, I "love to be talked to." This wonderful memento of my first days ends by saying, "That's about it, except to tell you he's the cutest, most adorable baby, and I'm sure you'll love and enjoy him as much as we did. P.S. He gets the hiccups frequently. It's nothing to worry about." And so, my life with my new family began.

That note has sat on my desk since my mom gave it to me some years ago. I look at it often, but don't often read it ... just look at it. It reminds me that, for the first month of my life, my family was a lady with nice handwriting. She loved and cared for me, bathed me, and talked to me. She kept me warm and safe and would get up every few hours each night so I wouldn't be hungry. She wasn't really my mom and she didn't give birth to me, but she was my family ... at least for a month.

My mom tells me that there was a hurricane on the day that lady with nice handwriting gave me to her and my dad. Apparently they had to pick me up on this day, or I'd go to the next family on the list. So, my new parents got in their car and braved a hurricane to make me their son.

I've never thought of my adopted parents as anything other than Mom and Dad. I never wondered about my birth parents growing up, although I did check into their background to try to understand my medical history when Kelly and I became parents. I've always known that I was adopted. When I was little, my mom would tell me, "Other people get whatever baby comes out, but we chose you." I think that she was worried that I would have a bad reaction to being adopted one day, but I never did.

My parents went on to have two more natural children, and I love my brothers with the same intensity that I imagine anyone else does. I've never been treated like an "outsider" or with jealousy, and, even though we don't see each other as often as I'd like, I love my brothers with all of my heart.

My father abandoned our family and my parents divorced when I was thirteen years old, but I never once considered that the man who walked out on us was anything but my father. Long after he had passed on, his departure remains one of the most devastating moments of my life. After he left, I would often in the middle of the night stand in our second-floor bathroom and look out on the road that led to our house. Even though I knew he wasn't coming back, I'd allow myself to feel excited when the lights from a random car brightened the street. In the brief moments between seeing the headlights and watching the car drive past our house, I'd imagine what our lives would be like again if he'd only change his mind and come home. Other nights, I'd sneak down to the living room and pull out the family portrait that my mom had taken down and stuffed into the back of a coat closet. It was in a big frame, and I'd sit with it on the couch until I felt better. Putting it back in the closet was always the worst part.

So much bad stuff in our lives came as a result of my father's inability to be a good husband. He cheated on my mom for years and then left us broke, both emotionally and financially. To make matters worse, even though we still lived in the same town, we almost never saw him. He quite literally threw us away. I realized when he died without ever really mending our relationship that he avoided us because of the shame he felt. My brothers and I lived our lives feeling abandoned, while our father lived his in a quiet agony of his own.

Unwittingly, his actions had a very unintended and delayed benefit for me, one that my children will enjoy for the rest of their lives. My dad and mom made the loving decision in 1971 to adopt a baby and give it a family life. The family that they built for me over the next thirteen years wasn't perfect, but it felt like it was to me. It turns out that, for all of our family's shortcomings, the simple act of wanting me was all that I needed. Being wanted is what family feels like to me. My father's leaving only served to cement my belief that family means more than anything else. It also taught me that there is no trauma greater to a child than to break up his or her family.

On the day of my thirteenth birthday, I got to pick the dinner menu because it was my day. We all ate together, and I remember exactly where I was sitting and how my dad looked when he excused himself to take a shower. He walked down the stairs a little while later with his hair still wet. He walked past me in the living room and continued through the house without saying a word. Then, I heard him walk out the back door. He never came back.

The lesson I learned that day was simple. I never wanted to be a man who could or would make his family feel as awful as he made us feel. People always talk about role models, and the common wisdom is that they should show you the right way to do things. My dad was my role model, for sure. However, I chose to see him as a cautionary tale instead of a how-to manual.

I made my family. Its existence is my doing. My wife wasn't looking to be married when I recognized that she was too good of a person to let her get away. Our son Cole and daughter Arden didn't, as kids will remind you, ask to be born. The four of us are together because of the decision that I made when I was knocked over by Kelly's beauty and charm. I pursued my wife, chasing her around for a full summer to get her to take me seriously. We've all made decisions since then that helped to shape this family, but it all began with me looking at a girl and saying, "Wow."

I know now as a grown man that there are moments when most adults think, "Maybe I should just go," but in my estimation there is no greater reward than family. There is no greener grass, no better life than the one that you can have with the family that you choose. Life is a journey, not a sprint, and not every moment will be packed with excitement. However, I do know that, if you stay until the end, the good parts will far outweigh the bad ones. My dad missed so many moments, and when I think of them I can't imagine not being with my kids on those days. When he cheated on my mom, he cheated us. But, worst of all, he cheated himself. I'm forty-one years old, and if I sit here and dwell even for a moment on the things that my dad and I never did together, I will cry like a baby.

Being a man doesn't mean cutting the lawn or fighting a guy for a parking spot. If you want to be a man, if you want your family to look at you and feel proud that you are their father, husband, and protector, all you have to do is support the first decision you ever made about them—the one that brought you all together when you saw your wife for the first time and thought, "Wow."

The Path to Parenthood Starts with Sex

In the spring of 1999, Kelly and I had been married for almost three years, and I was about to have my 29th birthday. Our blessed union had been fairly commonplace up until then. We were adjusting to being adults, living on our own, and working our first real jobs. We'd argue, have sex, see a movie, and do the rest of the stuff that we all do at this time in our lives. We were starting out well intended and full of life, but without an idea in the world about what we were doing, what any of it meant, or could one day become. We were married and in our twenties.

My path to becoming a stay-at-home dad started out innocently enough, and as each person's story about parenthood does ... with sex. On this magical day, there were no candles lit or frilly clothing like you read about in a romance novel. I wish I could say that my first child was born of a family plan, or even a romantic interlude, but the truth of the matter is that when you leave my wife alone for a while she gets lonely. Kelly had just spent the day alone in our tiny apartment because she was not feeling well and had taken the day off from work. The rest she got that day must have done her some good because she had just enough energy to accost me as I entered that evening after work. It was a tawdry affair, quick (no, not that quick), and to the point. The encounter happened with such surprise that elements of the encounter were forgotten ... and by that, I mean condoms. As I look back, I now realize that my son is only here today in the form that he is because Kelly had a cold. Had she gone to work that day he wouldn't be here, at least not this version of him. It's all so wonderfully random!

Some weeks later and far beyond the glow that we felt that day, the phone in my office rang. I was working as a graphic designer for a credit union at the time. I was able to get the position not because I had any training or background, but because I was the most computer-literate and creative person in the organization, and they were too cheap to pay anyone with real credentials.

When I answered the phone, it was Kelly. While I was happy to hear from her, it was the end of the day, not the normal time that we spoke to each other from work. She told me that she was calling from our apartment, and I became more confused. Kelly worked in the city and was never home this early. I asked her if everything was okay, and then she got quiet.

Kelly wasn't just calling me from our apartment, she was calling from the bathroom of our apartment, and she was holding a positive pregnancy test. The silence on the call following her announcement was taken as an indication that I wasn't happy, but in reality I was so much more than happy ... I was thrilled! I'd always wanted to have children, but I was unprepared for how the news that I would soon be a father would affect me. I immediately began to imagine all the things that I would need to do and instantly felt the pressure of another person's life depending on me. In those silent moments,

I quickly imagined my unborn child's life from that moment until its death, and I knew immediately that I was going to need to step up my game if that life was going to be one that was worth living.

When I finally spoke I was dumbfounded, and the sound of my voice apparently wasn't any comfort to poor Kelly. I was not able to convey my enthusiasm due to the immense amount of pressure that I suddenly felt. In the years following, I've had countless conversations with other men about this moment, and everyone agrees that you start feeling the weight of being responsible for your child the minute you learn that the child exists. The process isn't slow and building; you don't get time to get acclimated to the idea—it just hits you flat in the face.

I did my best to assure Kelly that I was excited despite my abnormally long period of silence, and then I rushed home to see her. What Kelly didn't know completely at the time was that she had just gotten knocked up by a guy who was perfectly suited to be a dad. I had always wanted children, and I put a lot of effort into figuring out which girls seemed like they'd be great moms, even when I was much younger. I knew that

Kelly was going to be the best mom that I could hope for even though I'm sure she wasn't as confident at the time. During my ride home, I thought about all the ways her personality was going to benefit our new baby, and I couldn't wipe the smile from my face. I married the smartest, prettiest, most wonderful girl, and she was going to be a fantastic mother, I just knew it.

About halfway through my ride home, I thought this exact thing: "Oh, no! Kelly can't stay home with the baby … her job is way better than mine." You see, I had a job, but Kelly had a career. She out-earned me by more than half, and her yearly increases were making mine seem nonexistent. I was instantly struck by the thought that we would have to use day care, which didn't seem ideal to me. Then, before I could delve too deeply into that problem, I realized that our apartment only had one bedroom and that we didn't live near our families anymore. The issues began to pile up in my head, and now I was battling with the logistical problems that a baby would bring. It had only been an hour since I found out that we were having a baby, and already it was feeling so new and unknown that I couldn't imagine that we would, in any way, be able to create a good life for it.

"This is what my mother meant," I thought. When I was a teenager she would say to me, "Wait until you see." I couldn't understand why with all of her life experience and knowledge all she could muster for advice was, "Wait until you see." Why didn't she tell me about the feelings and the pressure? Why didn't she articulate her experiences in a way that may have one day been of some help to me? Great, now I'm under pressure, mad at my mom, and trying to figure out where to put our baby while Kelly and I are working!

It is fair to say that, although I didn't have to carry the baby in my body, give birth, or be deluged with hormones that would make me act in ways that a young man couldn't imagine, this entire experience was making me nuts in less than an hour. I stood outside of our apartment door taking deep breaths, wanting to walk into the room like I had everything under control. I needed Kelly to feel like she made the right choice when she married me, because at that moment I wasn't too sure myself. The only comfort I felt was that I'd have nine months to figure everything out. What an idiot I was.

The Nine-Month Countdown

Just like that, we went from a carefree young married couple in our twenties to people who were about to have a baby. Suddenly we needed to know little things—at what hospital did we want to have the baby, did we want to know if the baby was a boy or girl, and many other questions that had seemed inconceivable only a few weeks prior.

Our "cute" apartment was now "small," and Kelly's metropolitan train ride into the city sounded like less fun with a bun in the oven. The lessons that we were about to learn were not fun, but they did help to get us ready to be parents. They would propel us into being adults, whether we liked it or not.

What I remember most about this time is the overall feeling that both of my feet were never planted firmly on the ground at the same time. I was forever off balance, like I had just forgotten something important. Every day seemed to bring a new experience that I didn't instinctually know how to handle.

New experience number one was a bit of a shocker. It seemed that by putting a baby in Kelly's belly I had unknowingly written myself an invitation to her OB/GYN appointments. In the past when one of these doctor's visits would come up, I would only be responsible for making the "wow, I'm sorry you have to do this" face as she left the apartment. Then I could play a video game or watch television while she was gone. I had, of course, accompanied her to other doctor's appointments—sick visits, eye exams, and the like—but these were waiting-room types of events. I wasn't ready for what a real OB appointment entailed.

My first time in the waiting room at the OB was weird, to say the least. I'm usually chatty even around strangers, but I found it difficult to speak to the people in this setting because I didn't know what circumstances brought them there. Many of the patients were pregnant, but others were just there for what I assumed was an annual physical. There is no polite conversation that begins, "So, your vagina huh?" I sat quietly. We filled out paperwork and did our best not to look as young as we were.

Soon, the nurse appeared at the doorway and called Kelly's name, and then she made eye contact with me. "Come on, Dad," she said.

It all started happening as I was still contemplating that the nurse had just called me Dad. Kelly had to get on a scale; then she peed in a cup and gave a blood sample. We weren't even in the exam room yet. I began looking around, and I was consumed with the thought that everyone was peeing and embarrassed by their weight. Pee, blood, and angry hormonal woman were all around me. Not one of them looked happy. I didn't think it could get any worse.

But it did ...

I don't know how to best say this, so I'm just going to blurt it out. If you have never seen, or had, a pelvic exam, let me tell you something—it's not how you imagine it. Maybe before I explain in detail about the exam, you should know this. I spent many months of talking and listening just to get Kelly to go on a date with me. Then I had to think up great places to take her on those dates and buy her flowers. I even made her chocolate chip cookies from scratch! I used the chocolate in the cookies to confuse her, and it worked just long enough for her to accept my invitation for a date. I spent an entire summer of my life getting Kelly to the point where giving me a kiss seemed like a good idea. It took great effort and a sincere amount of trickery, but I was able to confuse that poor girl into thinking that I was good enough to go out with her.

Now, a few short years later, here she is lying in a chair that looks like it was designed by a porn star. She was wearing the thinnest paper dress that I've ever seen, and she looked so scared, embarrassed, and helpless. Up until then, every moment that I had ever experienced with a naked girl was sexy. I remember looking at Kelly and thinking, "Fuck, getting her pregnant is ruining all of the fun that boobs bring to my life!"

When the doctor came into the room, it was impossible to not first notice his bow tie. He was a thin, quiet man, with no sense of humor that I could detect. He was polite and reserved and not terribly personable. After a little bit of chatter and a few answered questions, he put on some gloves, lubed up his hand, and then reached inside of my wife. I can't say that I was the most horrified person in the room, as I'm sure Kelly was none too happy, but holy crap, was I horrified! He went on to reach and feel, poke and squeeze, all while speaking to us about what he was doing like a tour guide.

Was this really what these appointments were like? I had always thought that women were exaggerating at least a little when they would talk about this stuff. I was stunned! Even though there was nothing even remotely sexual about this moment, I still had to watch a guy that I had just met three minutes before reach inside of my wife, and all I could think was, "He didn't even have to make her cookies." While Kelly was making her next appointment with the receptionist, I was still dazed.

Months later (or another way to think of it would be five pelvics later), we bought a small condominium. Kelly's pregnancy was coming along well, but her days at work were feeling long, and her commute was becoming taxing. She began to struggle. She was too tough and proud to ever say so, but I could tell. As we moved into our new home, decorated the baby's room, and went about living our lives, we patiently and nervously waited to meet our son. I remember that time fondly; we were making lists of baby names that we liked, picking out furniture and strollers, and looking for day care.

When I look back on the photos, I realize that I was unknowingly matching Kelly's weight gain almost pound for pound. I was happy, but the stress wasn't going away. In fact, it was growing. To this day, I owe the customer service person at Verizon Wireless an apology for how long, loudly, and unnecessarily harshly I yelled at him when Kelly couldn't get a cell connection from the train when she wasn't feeling well. It was my first time experiencing the helplessness that comes from being unable to help my family. It's a feeling that we would become far too familiar with in the future, but at this moment I didn't know how to handle the helplessness. I found it crushing, and I struggled to pull myself from under that feeling.

Some time in her third trimester Kelly got sick. She was experiencing a great deal of chest pain and was having trouble breathing. Eventually she had to undergo a test to make sure that she didn't have a pulmonary embolism (a blood clot in her lung), which could possibly kill her. When we asked if the test could hurt the baby, the doctor responded, "We hope not." At those moments, I found myself looking over my shoulder and wishing an adult would step up and make the difficult decisions. Suddenly, the questions weren't so simple. Now we were faced with real and lasting issues, ones with serious consequences. We finally decided that Kelly should get the test; there was no blood clot, and Cole was born a month later with the proper number of fingers and toes. Welcome to parenthood.

I Thought You Were Going to Keep Him Alive?

We aren't planners. I asked Kelly to marry me, and three weeks later we were married. Kelly spent one boring day alone in our apartment, and a week later she was pregnant. I assume you see the trend?

Sometime around the halfway point of gestation we began to wonder aloud what you do with a baby once it arrives. As far as we could tell, the baby-making pretty much happened on autopilot, but after he was born someone was going to have to, you know, keep him alive. The best we could figure that meant feeding, washing, and perhaps buying a cute pair of sunglasses or something. Who knew for sure?

I always wanted to be a father, but the truth is that

I only ever thought about it in simple terms. Baby comes out, it's cute, it poops, you wipe it off, repeat. Even though we hadn't yet given all of this baby stuff its due diligence, it did quickly dawn on us that the job would be a twenty-four-hour-a-day sorta thing and we already had jobs. We were sure that we couldn't pay for the baby's butt wipes and diapers if we didn't work, so I suggested kenneling the baby. Kelly told me that they called it day care when it's for humans, but that she thought I was on the right track. Then she also made a face that told me that she was considering that she might have married wrong.

Kelly worked far from our home and I was more local, so I took up the responsibility of visiting day care centers and reporting back to her. They all seemed pleasant enough. There were a few that I liked that were also close to our condo, so I began by visiting them. I called and made appointments, but I only kept the first one because after what I saw at that appointment, I couldn't bring myself to consider day care for another second.

You may think that I saw something egregious happen at that day care, or that the sight of fifty children all with runny noses scared me off, but it was quite the opposite. The building was new and the interior was wonderfully decorated. The children were happy and well-overseen; it was really rather warm and inviting. I took the tour and spoke to the people who worked there, and I was sure that this was the facility that we would end up choosing.

It was as I was standing by the front entrance and speaking with the director about pricing that I witnessed what pushed me over the edge. A father came through the door; he greeted the director and disappeared into a room just beyond where we were talking. A few minutes later he was wrestling with his son and trying desperately to get him to leave the room. When they finally emerged into the common space by the exit, the boy was visibly distressed because he didn't want to leave. At first I thought that it was because he was having fun or in the middle of playing with his friends, but I soon realized that what the boy desperately didn't want was to go with his father.

The boy, who appeared to be about four years old, told his dad that he wanted to stay with the teacher, and then he pulled away. He ran to the woman and held onto her leg for dear life. It wasn't the boy's actions or that he seemed to be more at home at the day care. It wasn't that he appeared to have a better bond with the teacher than with his father that broke my heart. It was the look on the man's face when he realized both these statements were true. I went home and told Kelly what I had witnessed, and I asked her to consider staying home with the baby when he was born.

Kelly laughed and laughed, not because her staying home was comical, but more due to the fact that my job didn't pay very well and hers did. Kelly had what you would call a career, while I had more of a job. Kelly had a degree, while what I had was really more of a diploma. Kelly had what you would call a bright future; again, I had a job. So, to be fair to Kelly, her laughing really was the correct response to my emotionally charged declaration that she should quit working and stay home with our yet-to-be-named bundle of joy.

I never expected what happened next. Kelly suggested that I quit my job and stay home. She said that she thought I'd make a great full-time dad and, to be honest, I did, too. We looked at the numbers, and it turned out that I made eighty dollars a month more than day care was going to cost. It seemed like a good idea, and we agreed to give it a try.

Now that I was going to be a stay-at-home dad, I was suddenly involved in decisions like strollers and other things that I had never imagined being a part of before we decided to try this role reversal. The experience has taught me one very important lesson—please pay close attention to this next bit. When your wife (or really any woman) asks for your opinion, she is just being polite. I may be overgeneralizing, but they don't care, even a little bit, what you think. And, to be honest, it's probably better that way. Nevertheless, there I was putting in my two cents on which bottles we should buy, breast-feeding accoutrements, car seats, and a host of other topics that I didn't know the first thing about and for which I had had zero instincts. Hindsight tells me that my wife had a vision. All I did while adding my thoughts and opinions was to ruin the experience for her.

She knew what she wanted the nursery to look like and what kinds of clothes the baby should wear. To be honest, I'm a guy, I didn't care at all, but what I did care about was my newfound sense of responsibility. As soon as we decided that I'd be taking care of the baby, I felt the need to be involved in things that I had never once considered in the past. All of a sudden, I had concrete opinions and needs regarding how and where things happened that most men don't even realize exist. I was slowly becoming a stay-at-home dad, and our role reversal was beginning to happen.

While I was busy adjusting to the idea of staying home, Kelly was trying to come to terms with the fact that she wasn't. I now understand that she felt a considerable amount of guilt about our decision. She was also contending with people's snide remarks about my masculinity and even a bit of jealousy on her part, all of which is understandable. She was having these feelings all while being inundated with pregnancy hormones to which her body was unaccustomed.

I handled the entire thing, I thought, very well. As most men do, I just went with the flow, joked my way through uncomfortable moments, and hyper-focused on my new responsibility. I was planning on being the world's best stay-at-home parent, and I didn't once consider any outside influences. See a problem, fix a problem. Nothing more manly than that!

Quitting My Job Was Like Starting Over

Growing up, I felt middle class. We weren't, but my parents did a very good job of making it feel like we were. My father was a working guy, and my mom kept the house and worked a part-time job about fifteen hours a week spread out over a few evenings.

No one ever once mentioned going to college to me. The conversation about school was always minimal and restricted to making sure that enough was done so that my parents wouldn't have to hear from our teachers. Academics and striving for more were never mentioned. My mom and dad had the same expectations for us as they had for themselves when they were our age—graduate from high school and get a job.

By the time administrators at my school noticed that I wasn't exactly on the fast track, it was too late for me; I was already following the example that had been set. Even though I always tested into advanced classes, my grades were average at best. I'd use my abilities to get by instead of achieving beyond the required basics. I was working toward graduation and nothing more. It's been well over twenty years since I graduated from high school, and I still believe that not taking my education seriously was the biggest personal mistake that I have made or likely will ever make.

It will come then as no surprise that I had to fight hard in the world as a young man to rise to the point where I could call myself a graphic designer. My early jobs were not exactly glamorous. I cut lawns, worked with photographic chemicals in a warehouse, ran an industrial steel saw, and jockeyed a register in a 7-Eleven.

When Kelly married me, I was mixing chemicals. The only good thing to come from that job was that the building was often empty, I had a key, and it was an exciting place to have sex. Since I didn't think that making love on a pallet of boxes was going to float Kelly's boat forever, I was always trying to improve my situation.

The one thing I had going for me was my mind, but I certainly didn't present to the outside world that I was any sort of an up-and-comer. However, I did continue to work hard and keep my eye out for opportunities that I could tackle with the tools that I possessed. I had a friend doing credit card collections who told me about an opportunity at her company. Getting that job was easy. The entire process was talking, and, as my gram would have said, I could talk "a blue streak." (I have no idea what that means.) I quickly excelled at persuading people to send a payment, and I was thrilled to be out of factories and in a clean shirt.

The aspect of the job that I couldn't bear was the emotional side. The one rule taught to debt collectors is "assume everyone is lying." You can't ask people to send money after they've told you about a spouse's illness or that they hope to have enough to make a payment if they can sell enough chickens this week unless you think they aren't telling you the truth. People have to disconnect themselves from their souls to do that job, and, the better I became at it, the less I could respect myself. So when the next opportunity came along, I took it.

That next job was doing private collections for a credit union. But they saw their customers as an extension of a family, so these "collection calls" were more like friendly phone reminders. I'd call the same few hundred people every month, we'd chat, and then I'd gently remind them to send a payment. Bottom line, it wasn't collections, and I was happier for a while, but I always expected more from myself.

When I heard that the credit union had lost its graphic designer, I swooped in to get the position. How did I get a job for which I had absolutely no qualifications or training? Simple—I talked my way into it. Then I hustled to learn the position before they realized that I didn't know what I was doing. I must have done well enough, because I held that position for a number of years and by all accounts did a fine job.

From the time that I graduated from high school until the day that I handed in my resignation at my design job, I had a bunch of crap jobs. I worked at times for less than four dollars an hour, in the searing heat and the insane cold. I almost cut my finger off, spent a year feeling terrible about every word that I spoke, and created thousands of interest-rate pamphlets. Every moment at those jobs reminded me of how I had squandered my time in high school and screwed up by never seriously considering that I should go to college.

It wasn't until we made the decision that I would stay at home with our son that I realized that my journey through my hodgepodge of a resume was my education, and that my time in these different lines of work had prepared me for my real job. I had jobs that taught me patience and one that showed me that my surroundings were never as bad as they could be. I learned how to play at being professional and that I had limits to what I would do to make money. I finally felt qualified for a job that I was taking. Even if I wasn't, I wouldn't have to talk my way into it—I was sleeping with the human resources person.

The most difficult moment in leaving my career to become a stay-a-home wasn't the quitting or the un-certainty. I didn't really even worry too much about the money aspect. I was excited to start my new job and only concerned about one thing. I thought back on the journey that I had had to take to go from a convenience store clerk to a graphic designer. Every time I made a change, I had asked someone to trust that I could do the job that they desperately needed to have done. What would happen to me if staying home didn't work out? Would I fall all the way back to cutting lawns? Oh, God, I couldn't work at 7-Eleven again! What would happen to me if I got thrown back in the working world?

Starting a new job is always unnerving. Even if you have a perfect skill set, you still walk in one day as a complete stranger to the process. Where do you park? Sit? Whom do you have to impress? What time is lunch? Can you do this? We all have the same concerns on day one, doesn't matter if you are making the fries, running the world, or raising a baby. Everything is new, and you have to find out how you fit in.

What you may not realize is that when you redefine the responsibilities of your marriage in this way you cease, in your partner's eyes, to be the person that you were the day before. Now you are the one charged with raising your children, and your partner expects that you'll do that job well. Not only because your partner wants the best for your child, but because they are losing their shot at being that person in your family. You are taking on a responsibility that doesn't offer a second chance and where failure carries great consequence. I knew my wife was watching me, and not wanting to let her or our son down was the largest pressure that I had ever faced. I would spend the next ten years trying to find a balance between being me and the person that I imagined my family needed me to be.

A Typical Day at My Office

7:30 AM Rounded up dirty clothes and put in a load of laundry.

8:00 Struggled to get Cole out of bed.

8:41 Cole prepped for his day and on the bus.

8:50 Woke up Arden (my second child—more about her later).

9:00 Oh my God, I have to pee! So does our dog Indy, so let him outside instead. Feed him.

9:05 Tested Arden's blood glucose, discuss breakfast carbs, dose insulin. (More to follow on Arden's diabetes.)

9:08 Explained to Arden that Kelly is still her mom and my wife even if she loses her job (no idea how that thought got into her head).

9:10   Visited with Arden's hamster Rudolph at Arden's request.

9:15   Prepped kitchen floor to be cleaned.

9:22   Finally got to the bathroom.

9:25   Made breakfast for Arden.

9:30   Almost got my pants on, still in a pair of shorts.

9:32   Refilled napkin dispenser (that was bugging me).

9:35   Cleaned a candleholder that had wax all over it.

9:40   Loaded dishwasher.

9:50   Laundry at top of stairs to basement.

9:55   Cleaned up the computer cords that Kelly abandons every night when she is finished with her laptop.

9:57   How did this bat get here? Took Cole's bat bag to his room.

10:00   Looked at the dirty laundry in Cole's room that I didn't know about. Took to basement.

10:05	Another load of laundry.
10:09	Arden wants a banana.
10:12	Got Arden an apple because the banana "wasn't tasting right."
10:15	Cleaned powder room; washed floor, toilet, sink. Watered plants and refilled toilet paper.
10:30	Vacuumed.
10:45	Cleaned the dog's ears. Gross!
10:50	Stripped bed sheets.
10:55	More dirty laundry to the basement.
11:00	Put Kelly's shoes and headbands away. (This is a full-time job.)
11:10	Made iced tea, got hungry, and tried to make something for myself.
11:12	Washed the dog's bowls and fed Indy while I waited for the microwave.
11:13	Tried to eat, but diabetes needed something.
11:20	Made tea with Arden.
11:25	Arden and I put candle wax on our fingers; that was fun.
11:28	Dog had to pee again, taking forever!
11:40	Bathroom break, able to read 2.5 pages of

the book I'll never get through.

11:48   Telemarketer.

11:50   Shower for Arden, dressed, brushed hair and teeth.

11:58   Thought about Arden's blood glucose and worried because of last test. Talked about lunch. Petted Indy.

12:05 PM Hug-wrestled with Arden, cuddled, talked about Mousey's dog's dental habits. Mousey is Arden's invisible mouse friend. Mousey has a dog, and he apparently doesn't brush often.

12:25   Talked with Mrs. Hanson on Arden's 911 phone (recorded voice on a play phone). Was able to schedule story time with make-believe lady on pretend phone.

12:40   Dog needed to go out again. Let him out without collar by mistake, uggghhh! Finally got dog back in.

1:05   Tested Arden. Gave shot. Set up Arden with her craft. Switched over laundry. Put in another load. Brought up ton of clean laundry.

1:15   Wanted to fold laundry, but now is a good time for my shower because Arden's blood glucose is in a stable range and the dog is lying down. Almost got in shower ... dog jumped on sofa. Cleaning mud from ottoman.

1:26   Out of shower and dressed. The next three hours go on like this: play time, FedEx, called school, diabetes, dog, laundry, dishes, garbage, doctor's appointments.

4:00   Cole arrives home from school. Now it's make dinner, homework, sibling fights, clean up from dinner, more garbage to the curb, spills, laundry, phone calls, and it doesn't stop.

7:05   I decided that I no longer want to track my day and I stopped making the list, but the day kept going.

Being a stay-at-home parent is a series of never-ending tasks, and most days go like the one you just read about. Much as in the workplace, there are politics to navigate, schedules to keep, deadlines to hit, stress, pressure, guilt—and you never feel like you are getting ahead.

I didn't initially expect that I would become more emotional than I already was, but this job will change you. There is something about being around children twenty-four hours a day that makes a person feel more intensely, love harder, and protect fiercely. You cannot be with your children and give them the parent/child relationship that they need and deserve if you are in any way walled off or disconnected from the basic feelings that make us all human.

Most moms whom I meet have this "ability" from the moment their first child is born, sometimes sooner. If you are a man raising children, I think that you need to purposely deactivate the mechanism that many of us have that says, "Men don't cry." If you can do that, I promise that your life will be filled with the most touching and wonderful memories, that your days will overflow with boundless joy. If you can bring yourself to feel on that level, you'll learn what the mothers of the world know instinctually ... there is a lifetime full of happiness in your children's eyes. Once you've let your guard down you'll begin to see the pauses in between the busy moments, and you'll enjoy every last second of their personal discoveries as they grow into adults.

To Think I Was Worried About Baby Vomit

The day that Cole was born

I made three mistakes. The stories of those mistakes are burned into my memory, and I have no choice but to remember them as my wife brings them up almost all the time.

Mistake number one would have easily been avoided by the man that I am today. There is no way that I now would have believed that Kelly *really* wanted me to take a break during her long wait for our son and go to the cafeteria for a snack. The me that I am today is too savvy. He would know that no matter what Kelly said, I should never leave the delivery room, no matter how many hours we were trapped in there or how hungry

I was. Poor twenty-nine year old Scott took her at her word and then did something that will never be forgotten in our home—I had a few Doritos that left my breath smelling very "nachoee."

Soon after I returned from my nosh, Kelly was ready to deliver, and it was time for me to make mistake number two. Much of our family was in and out of the delivery room that day, and, when push came to shove, it got a little hectic in the room. Both of our mothers were there when the baby began to come, and it never occurred to me to ask my mom to leave the room when the birthing started. I'll never know which mistake bothers Kelly more. Was it that I stood by her face trying to calm her with the dopey phrases that I learned in birthing class, all the while unknowingly breathing a nauseating nacho cheese odor into her face? She does still seem to delight in telling the nacho breath story, but I think she's more annoyed that my mom saw her vagina.

My third mistake doesn't get spoken about as often, but it's the one that I regret the most. Later in the evening as we were hanging out for the first time as a family in the hospital room, I fell to sleep in Kelly's bed and never woke up. She slept the entire night in an uncomfortable reclining chair while I rejuvenated myself in her bed. I feel terrible to this day about that, and thinking about it now causes me to wonder how many other stupid things I've done over the years.

It took a few hours for Cole to pink up after he was born. Kelly was given a narcotic during birth that we never would have agreed to if we had been older and surer of ourselves. The drug (and my Doritos breath) made Kelly nauseous during most of the day, which was terrible, and it also made Cole come out a little, let's say, high. A few hours later when he was able to leave the nursery, the nurse brought him to us. This was the first moment of real terror that I felt as a new parent. The hours since Cole's birth were full of phone calls and taking people to the nursery window to see Cole. None of it was real yet, but it was about to be.

When the nurse came into our room she told us where we could find the diapers and wipes, asked where we wanted the bassinet, and then began to walk out. When I saw her leaving the room I panicked and yelled, "Where are you going?" Then I spoke one of the most honest sentences of my life: "Look, you don't know us, but I'm almost positive that you will be breaking a law leaving him here; I can't promise that we can keep him alive." She smiled and said that we'd be okay, but I wasn't kidding. It turned out that I couldn't have been more wrong. I felt in control almost immediately, and I learned that what didn't come naturally would be perfected with practice.

Cole's stomach was sensitive for the first six or so months of his life. When we fed him a bottle, we'd have to hold him perfectly still for a while afterward or he'd vomit up the entire bottle. I want to try to describe what it feels like to have a bottle of recently consumed formula vomited back onto you. I can still feel how warm it was and so thick, though the smell should not be under-appreciated. The mixture of the rancid smell with the warm thick liquid was just terrible enough to make you forget how expensive the mix was as it splashed about on everything in its path. I knew that I was a pro on the day that I didn't rush to wipe myself off after an attack. I was, however, an amateur compared to Kelly. She once held it together after Cole vomited into her open mouth. That little baby vomited in stores, all over Kelly at a funeral, in the car, anywhere really, he just puked and puked for months. We had those vomit rags on every flat surface in our condo and you still couldn't get to one fast enough when you needed it. Then one day he just stopped and never did it again.

Much like the vomit, most of the things that I initially worried about turned out not to be issues at all. Vomit, poop, finding a schedule, not dropping him— all of that stuff was easy. Though getting peed on was unsettling in the beginning, and I did freeze for a second the first time I miscalculated with the wipe and got poop on my hand. However, none of it seemed to really matter or affect me the way I worried that it would.

The benefit from being that close to your children right from the start is that you fall in love with them in a way that you might not be able to if you aren't their mother. Moms have it almost right away. They fall in love with their children in a way that most men can't imagine. I'm one of the lucky men that get to experience what it means to have the feeling of a mother's love.

Watch other people when you are out. Men tend to

rub their kids on the head to show affection, while moms put their arms around them. Woman linger longer; men are generally in and out of loving moments quickly. Men rarely kiss their kids after they are a few years old; women need to be told by their teenagers that kissing is over now. I know that being that openly loving can feel awkward to guys, but I am so happy that I have that kind of relationship with my kids.

It's going to be your inclination to worry about the vomit, or how to pay for college when your baby is born, but I really suggest that you focus on breaking the old ideas of how a man behaves with his children. I hug my kids every day, and we linger for a few moments. We close our eyes and try to melt into one another.

I've noticed that many fathers find their sons before they participate in a sporting event. Cole plays so much baseball, and I've heard the other guys offer last-minute advice or attempt to speak words of motivation to their boys. If you ever see me in those moments, it will appear that I am doing the same, but I don't just tell Cole to keep his weight back when he hits. I also bend down and whisper, "I love you." And, if his friends aren't watching,

I give him a kiss. I know how strange that may seem to you if you are a man reading this, but before you pass judgment, know this: Cole is halfway through his season and about to begin playing for the sixth straight year on our town's all-star team. He leads off on two teams and his batting average is .476. "Go get 'em" may be classic, but "I love you" works amazingly well, too!

I Only Dropped Him Once

By my count, I've come close to breaking, losing, or otherwise ending Cole's life three times so far in the twelve years that he's been alive. When you take into consideration that I've dropped or misplaced my iPhone at least that many times this week, I don't think three times is all that bad. The fact that I've come close to accidentally ending the boy isn't what makes these stories worth telling—it's more about the how.

Break: The first time that I almost killed Cole scared the crap out of me and tested my soccer skills, which I freely admit to not having had in my life before or since this moment. One Saturday afternoon Kelly took Cole with her for a bubble bath—he must have been about nine months old at the time. They played together with boats, stuck foam letters to the tile walls, and piled bubbles as high on their heads as they could. When they finished, Kelly asked me to take Cole to his room and get him dressed so that she could stand up and use the shower. I laid an adult-sized towel on this wonderfully thick and woolly rug that we had in that bathroom. I dried him off as we played for a few minutes. Then I wrapped him in his towel to keep him warm (how great is it to wrap a little baby in a towel after a bath?) and we went to his room to choose an outfit from the closet.

He wasn't slippery or in any way difficult to hold as I stood by the closet trying to decide among the nine thousand outfits that we received as gifts. His towel was around his back, but below his shoulder and wrapped around his little body just so. I had him on my left side; his butt was about even with my forearm, which was slightly above my waist; and I was pressing his body firmly to mine just as I had done countless times before. I only turned my head for a moment to choose an outfit. As I turned back to Cole with a hanger in my right hand, he bent his legs at the knees, planted his feet firmly into my side, and pushed as hard as he could, as if it was his intention to do a back flip and land on his feet. He pushed hard, so hard that his body did in fact flip back and out of my grasp.

The next few seconds seemed to happen on two different planes of existence. The physical aspects of this event happened at full speed. Cole bending his legs, the push, the flip, and the rapid descent all took two seconds. It happened in the blink of an eye. In my head, however, time seemed to be still. I experienced more thoughts in those few seconds than I ever could imagine possible. I turned toward Cole as he fell and in an instant saw that two things were true—I couldn't catch him, and he was going to fall directly onto the top of his head with the full weight and force of his body driving down from above. I had the conscious thought that he was going to die if I didn't do, not just something, but the right thing.

So I kicked Cole in the side of his head purposely so that he wouldn't fall straight down on his head and neck, but I did it with a gentle ease that still to this day surprises me. The motion of my foot and leg sort of just caught him. I'm finding it difficult to describe, but I didn't kick him with any force; there wasn't a collision between my foot and his head. They just gently met, and the motion of my leg turned his body ninety degrees, and he fell gently onto his side.

Initially he didn't cry, and it's possible that he might never have had I not screamed for Kelly so loudly. She called from the bathroom and asked what was wrong, but I couldn't answer her. I kept repeating, "Come here fast!" Cole began to cry as Kelly made her way to us. I couldn't bring myself to touch him, literally believing that I had caused him a lasting injury. When Kelly crossed the threshold of the room, Cole was lying on the floor crying, and I was standing above him in shock.

"What happened?" she cried.

I replied softly, "I dropped him … I'm sorry."

This marks the first time that I really understood the fact that Kelly and I were only married, that our connection was based on a decision. Though we had decided to be together, we weren't bonded in the same way that we were individually to Cole. The protective feeling that we each had, the one that would allow us to do anything to protect him, didn't extend to each other.

I never imagined that would be the case, but this moment taught me that it certainly was.

If Cole was seriously hurt I was never going to forgive myself, but in that instant I knew for sure that the punishment that I would serve to myself wouldn't hold a candle to the animosity that Kelly would have toward me if I had injured our baby. Thankfully, he was fine, not a scratch, not a bruise, not even a bump. As I looked into Kelly's eyes I could see that if he was indeed seriously injured, we were finished. I don't think she or I, for that matter, at that point in our lives, could have forgiven the other in a situation like that, accident or not. I hope that I never find out if our relationship, now more mature, could handle such a thing.

Lose: The day that I almost lost Cole showed me that there was nothing that I wouldn't do to protect him. I'm going to put Cole's age when this happened at around two and a half years. We went to a Walmart-like store to buy paper products for the house—napkins, toilet paper, and such. Before we did the shopping, I took Cole to the toy section and let him look around. We weren't buying anything on this day. The browsing was part of my concept that it would be possible to raise children who didn't ask for a gift every time they found themselves in a store if we practiced wanting something and not always getting it.

The toy section had about five aisles—each was made up of two approximately fifteen-foot lengths. So it was fifteen feet of toys, cross the main path, and another fifteen feet of toys, five times over. Cole and I were walking around, trying out the toys and talking about which ones he might want to ask for when Christmas rolled around. Suddenly he got a burst of energy and decided to run up and down the aisles. He wasn't very fast, so I chased him a little in one direction, and then I'd pass and cut him off. He'd turn around and go the other way; it was a few moments of fun. The last time he got to the path in between the aisles I grabbed him around the waist and said, "Gotcha." Then I spun him around and faced him the other way. He smiled at me so big and then got this mischievous look on his face before beginning to back away from me. I let him go almost the entire length of the fifteen feet before I pretended to be coming after him. When I began to move toward him, he turned the corner at the end of the aisle to get me to chase him. I took one big step to make him think I was coming and then turned around. I was going to try and scare him by unexpectedly showing up in the next aisle and blocking his path. I turned and took a few steps, bound around the corner, and he wasn't there. I thought he must have outsmarted me and doubled back, so I went back to the aisle that we had just left, but he wasn't there either. Then I began to quickly move up and down the aisles frantically searching for Cole, but he was gone. Gone! I called his name, no response. Called again, "Cole!?" Nothing.

My mind immediately jumped to the idea that someone might have grabbed him, and I felt like I had only seconds before he would be taken from that store and I'd never see him again. "Run to the exit!" my brain screamed at me but there was more than one exit. What if I picked the wrong one? So I did the only thing that made sense, the only thing I could think of. I screamed at the top of my lungs. Screamed loudly and clearly without a moment's hesitation.

"I lost my son ... he's little and wearing an orange

shirt and blue pants." I listened for a moment, but the din that exists in every large space when filled with people didn't change. All I could hear were the muffled sounds of shoppers talking to each other. "Listen to me!" I shouted. "Stop what you are doing and look for my son ... everyone, orange shirt, blue pants, brown hair, light skin ... LOOK AROUND—NOW!"

Silence blanketed the store after I yelled the second time. I stood motionless in the silence and waited for someone to relieve my anguish, but no one spoke. My eyes filled up, my chest felt like someone had reached down my throat and grabbed my heart. The store and its aisle suddenly felt endless to me as I tried to imagine which way Cole could have gone. I was about to panic when a voice rang out. "I have him," a woman yelled. "He's here." The enormity of that moment lasted maybe a minute, and then I grabbed Cole and hugged him like I hadn't seen him in twenty years. Cole was unaware of any problem and the very kind woman who found him said, "It's okay, he's fine ... great idea yelling like that." She smiled and walked away as the din enveloped the store once again.

Otherwise ending: In December of 2008, I found myself with an offer to attend Barack Obama's inauguration ceremony. I was able to get four tickets. Not general admission to the ceremony, either; we were going to have chairs on the Capitol lawn. Arden was young, so she couldn't go, and Kelly offered to stay home with her, knowing that I'd enjoy the experience more than she probably would. I invited my brother Brian and our longtime friend Aly, leaving the last ticket for Cole if he wanted it. Cole was eight years old when January rolled around. He couldn't seem to make a decision as to whether or not he wanted to come with us, but I never offered the ticket to anyone else. Just before bedtime on the eve of our departure, Cole came to me and said that he wanted to come to D.C. with us. We woke up extra early the next day and went to our local hunting and fishing superstore to buy Cole a jacket, gloves, and the rest of the accessories that he would need to withstand prolonged exposure to the extreme cold.

We spent that night at Aly's aunt's place just outside of D.C. The next morning we woke up before the sun, bundled ourselves up, and made our way to the train that would take us to the "Nation's Front Yard." The crowds were massive, unlike anything that I've ever seen. No sporting event or theme park could have prepared us for what millions of people gathered in the streets feel like. There were so many people that the seemingly simple act of crossing the street or walking out of the Metro station became an exercise in critical thinking and physical determination. We eventually found the line for our entrance at 7:30 in the morning. It was almost eight blocks long, and each person in it was shoulder-to-shoulder with at least three others.

The cold was remarkably piercing. I found myself hoping that we would get through security quickly so that perhaps the excitement of the day would provide us with some artificial warmth as we waited at our seats for the festivities to begin. Politics aside, I was very excited for Cole to be present at such a historic occasion for our country. Of the millions of gatherers in attendance, I only saw maybe a handful of children Cole's age. I felt very strongly that this day could create a lasting memory for Cole and that he would leave the Capitol with a story that few other people his age would ever be able to claim. That's how I felt at 7:30, anyway.

At half past noon, I wasn't so hopeful. Making it past the security gate now seemed unlikely. We had traveled baby step by baby step for the last five hours, and even though we could now see the gate, it still looked to be farther away than we could traverse in thirty minutes. I began to feel sad. I had gotten Cole so close to this, and he was going to leave completely disillusioned and unfulfilled. I began to ask myself why I hadn't left earlier in the morning; should I have been less cattle-like in my acceptance of the line; what could I have done to secure a better outcome for us? I felt like I should have tried something different. We trudged along with a defeated look on our faces, and I began to talk to Cole about managing our expectations, wanting to ready him for the letdown that seemed to be just around the bend.

The first five hours and fifteen minutes that we spent in this thick line taught me a valuable lesson. I saw that people could get along very nicely even in unpleasant situations, that you could put strangers in a tough spot, and they could respond with kindness and grace. It was uplifting and a frequent topic among our group as we passed that time. The lesson I learned in the final fifteen minutes before the inauguration began stood, however, in stark contrast. At 12:45 PM, our little group was about forty yards from the gate. The line had devolved into a gathering, a mass of bodies all trying to break the bottleneck that had formed when the order of the line ceased to exist. I looked around and began to take stock of the faces in the crowd. Displeasure was growing quickly; something bad was going to happen.

I wiggled next to my brother Brian, who is much taller and bigger than I am and whispered in his ear. "This is going to fall apart really fast. These people are beginning to realize that they aren't going to make it through in time. We have to protect Cole when things get nuts."

He nodded to me and looked around for somewhere to hide Cole. He understood now, as I did, that there was no moving in any direction but the one that the collective chose. We were stuck in the center of thousands of people and at the mercy of the tide. A moment later a voice came over the loudspeaker at the Capitol. It sounded farther away than I had expected it to. I don't know exactly what was said, but the crowd heard that the ceremony would be starting shortly. That news started a crack in the dam. Unrest flooded the area, and the polite tones of conversation turned on a dime. Now there was grumbling and complaining, and I knew what was coming next. I grabbed Brian again and said, "Someone is going to yell, and then the shit is going to hit the fan. We have to surround Cole and try to keep the pressure of the crowd off of him."

And then it happened as if on cue: "LET US IN!"

My eyes locked with Brian's. "Here we go," I said. I was scared for Cole, Brian looked frightened, and I couldn't even turn my shoulders to see Aly. We each put a hand on Cole's shoulder and grabbed a fistful of his jacket. With that, the eight blocks of people behind us seemed to all push at once. It was terrifying. We tried our best to keep moving toward the opening in the gate, and we were making out pretty well until we smacked into a ten-foot length of discarded metal fence that earlier in the day must have been part of a cattle chute. This section, however, was still standing, and it was blocking our way. We were stuck, but at least the crowd was trying to go around us now instead of through us. I asked Cole if he was okay and told him that I was sorry, but it looked like ten feet from the gate was as close as we would get to the inauguration. I had given up.

Cole looked at me and, for the first time, he looked sad, too. His gaze broke my heart the rest of the way— I had let him down. I had built this moment up for weeks, spoken about being present for history, and after all of the effort we put in, ten feet and a metal gate had stolen our chance to be a part of this historic day.

As it turns out, all our situation needed was a child's perspective. I'm going to tell you what happened next without even a hint of exaggeration. I couldn't comprehend it as it happened, so I'll understand if you have trouble believing. Cole looked into my eyes and said, "We aren't really going to get this close and stop, are we?"

I said, "I don't want to, but we are stuck. I can't move."

Cole looked at me like he was meant to take over the situation and asked, "Can you jump this thing? … cause I can!" Then he threw himself over the four-foot-tall fence. I jumped right behind him. I looked back for Brian and Aly, but the crowd seemed to have swallowed them up. Civility and a sense of personal safety left me when I saw the security gate now so close in front of us that it seemed possible to reach.

I wedged myself past Cole and screamed, "Hold onto the back of my coat … don't let go and run when I do." I pushed and clawed my way through the last few feet of humanity in front of us, determined to get Cole to the Capitol lawn. Rough jackets and zippers scratched at my face, and I could only see what was right in front of me. I thought for a moment that we couldn't make it; that's how tightly pressed together our bodies were. But I pushed and twisted and drove my legs, motivated by Cole's small hands on my back.

We shot through the edge of the crowd and through the gate with such force that our momentum nearly knocked us down when we ceased to experience any resistance. I don't know what I looked like, but Cole's face was wearing a smile like I'd never seen. We rushed through the metal detectors and met on the other side.

"Where's Uncle Brian and Aly?" Cole asked, as he was being checked by the security officer.

"I don't know, but we have to go ... we'll find them later," I said, all the while thinking that we wouldn't see them again until we got back to the house that night. I looked up and came to the realization that the damn security checkpoint was four blocks from the Capitol. A voice on the loudspeaker announced, "Five minutes." I grabbed Cole and we took off running.

Needless to say, our seats were taken when we got to the lawn. Actually, I think they were, but we couldn't get within a hundred yards of them, so I can't be sure. Our new problem was that there were so many people overflowing into the area around the Capitol that every square inch that had a line of sight to the podium was occupied. There was no more persevering, no last fence to hop, and I wasn't about to push through another person. We were going to have to stand next to a bushy pine tree and just listen to the moment. Being here was going to have to be enough, because we weren't going to see anything. I bent down to apologize to Cole. He told me that he felt like we made it, that this spot was good enough for him. I didn't feel the same. This day needed one more creative thought, one more rally cry, one last fence needed to be jumped over, and I found it when I looked over Cole's shoulder.

"Climb into the tree," I said softly, not wanting to give my great idea to anyone else. "Climb, I'll be right behind you … try and get far enough off the ground to see over the crowd and then make your way to the other side of the tree."

Cole and I watched President Obama take his oath of office while we were stuffed into a pine tree on the Capitol lawn. We were frozen, tired, and about eight hours past needing a bathroom break. Everything that could have, and ten things I didn't imagine, went wrong that day. In the span of twenty minutes, I went from being truly positive that I had brought my son to Washington, D.C., so that he could be trampled to death on the street to experiencing one of the most perfect moments of my life. I have a great picture of Cole in the tree.

When the ceremony was over, we climbed down and I somehow saw my brother and Aly standing in the distance. Brian was hugging a complete stranger. The moment was so powerful, he told me later, that he and the gentleman who stood next to him just instinctually hugged one another.

As a parent, you are going to screw up more times than you'll be able to remember as you raise your children. You may drop them, lose them for a few minutes, or make a decision that comes close to being the worst of your life. However, if you just keep moving forward, ask for help when you need it, never give up, and scream at the top of your lungs once in a while, things should turn out fine almost every time. Maybe not as you pictured ... but pretty damn good.

A Little Help from My Favorite Books

In the early days, weeks, and months of Cole's life, everything I did felt like it was for the first time. From the smallest almost ignorable moments to the big in-your-face situations, none of what I was doing felt familiar and each failure seemed to compound the last. As the weight of my perceived failures became overwhelming, I reached out to some of my favorite authors for help.

One of my favorite books, *Outliers: The Story of Success* by Malcolm Gladwell, suggests that a person requires ten thousand hours of practice to become proficient at something. Though the concept of ten thousand hours didn't hit my radar until both of my children were already here, it helped me to develop a sincere appreciation for taking my time and leaning on love, understanding that with practice it would get better.

Another of my favorite books would help me through a tough time. My adventure began when Cole was around a year old. The tightness in my back began soon after Cole and I dropped Kelly off at the train station that day, and it progressively worsened over the next few hours. What began as a tight muscle in my back quickly turned into a debilitating spasm that left me lying flat on the floor and trying to parent a baby without the use of my legs. I was incapacitated, and Cole was crawling around and over me. He was acting as if our living room was a giant Thomas the Train set and I was the bridge. I grabbed another favorite book of mine, *Healing Back Pain: The Mindbody Prescription* by Dr. John Sarno. I tried tips from the book to relax for over an hour, but relief wasn't coming.

An earlier reading of Dr. Sarno's book had taught me that many, if not all, of my back ailments were stress related. His lessons had kept me free of back pain–related issues until this day. Dr. Sarno writes, and I believe, that when your stresses become too much for you to handle and you aren't dealing with them properly, your brain gives you something else to think about. He believes that the unseen damage that comes with living with constant stress is far more damaging than pain in your back, neck, or head. His book taught me how to bring those stresses to the forefront of my thinking so that I could deal with them and release the pain.

In the past, however, my issues had been far less complex. In those days, I was simply a young man disappointed with his job and worried about money. It was easy for me to identify triggers such as those, but this incident proved different. Now I was a man in his late twenties who had just had a baby, quit his job, and given over his life to caring for someone else. I wasn't sleeping or eating properly, and everything I did was new. To complicate matters further, the person I was doing it all for couldn't speak, so I couldn't ask if I was doing any of it correctly. I had given up my income, and even though she never once mentioned money, I suddenly felt like I had to ask my wife if I could buy even the smallest item.

On the other side, Kelly was now living with the

immense pressure of being the only person earning an income. Everything in our lives had changed, and most of it seemed to be for the worse. The only bright spot that I could identify some days was Cole. Of course there were many more positives, but change has a way of making you look at the negative.

I eventually gave up on the idea that I was going to be able to get up off of the floor on my own. Since Cole certainly wasn't going to be any help, I called Kelly, and she made the long trip home after only being at work for a couple of hours. She had to take a train and then a cab to get to our home, and when she arrived I was still lying on the floor. I was embarrassed and in pain. Kelly looked down at me with such concern and love that I didn't feel judged at all. She helped me up and into a warm bath, comforting and consoling me along the slow walk to the bathroom. I'll never forget what she said to me when I finally got into the tub.

Kelly didn't have the experience that I did with Dr. Sarno, so she was a bit wary of the idea that visualizing the things that cause you stress could relieve actual physical pain. Still, she looked me in the eye and said,

"You're just freaking out because everything is so different. You're going to be a great dad, and all of this is going to feel like you've been doing it your entire life very soon." Then she assured me that she was going to take care of Cole while I did "my trick" to loosen up my back. "You'll be fine in a few hours," she said, as she closed the bathroom door. "Call if you need anything."

"My back is not hurt, I'm fine. I'm worried about (fill in the blank) …" That's the phrase that I use when I have a tight back, stiff neck, or other unexplainable aliment that is keeping me from enjoying my day. An hour later, armed with the knowledge that my wife, pardon the pun, had my back, I emerged from that tub free of the pain that slammed me to the floor six hours earlier. Something else happened that day, something that set me on the path that I find myself on to this day. I realized how much being a good dad meant to me. I was so subconsciously worried that I was going to be a crappy dad that the concern became physically debilitating.

While I thank Dr. Sarno when his techniques help me, it wasn't just the visualization that pulled me from my own mind's grip. Kelly's words fell over me like warm caramel on ice cream. They made me feel protected. Knowing that she believed in me was all I needed to move forward. Equally important to me was that I figured out that I wasn't just staying home with our son because my career wasn't as hopeful as Kelly's. I was choosing the path, and I wanted to walk it the best that I could. When I think back on that day, I really believe that I was reacting to the fear that I did not want to become my dad.

That's the day that I realized that I was a stay-at-home dad for all of the right reasons. Even though I didn't know how to put the bottle nipples into the dishwasher the first time that I tried, I'd figure it out. I stopped thinking about my days like someone from the outside looking in and I threw myself into my new life completely. I wasn't close to having my ten thousand hours in yet that day, but I knew for sure that my attitude was going to have a lot to do with how I lived those hours as they happened. Since then, I've dropped my ego, put away my silly pride, and picked up a dishcloth, and I couldn't be happier that I did.

By the way, none of this applies to the laundry. Laundry still sucks. Buddha would bitch about doing the laundry.

Lunch with the Lions

People have children for many different reasons, but when those children arrive, being a parent is a task for which few of us are prepared. We all have an image in our minds about what parenthood will be like. We think about perfect babies and strong grown children. In our minds, our children are always intelligent, kind, and successful. No one pictures his or her child as rude, uncultured, and misbehaving. Not one parent lifts a newborn baby for the first time and thinks, "I bet this kid turns out to be a hot mess." We all imagine the mountaintop for our children—President of the United States, a captain of industry, maybe a doctor. The ultimate question is: how do you maximize their potential and give them the best shot at becoming a well-balanced person without completely screwing them up?

In my opinion, the key to unlocking your child's potential is exposure. If it's your goal to raise a child to be just like you, then there isn't much to do. On the other hand, if you want to really find out what makes your children tick, expose them to the world. Watch what makes them smile, and let them run in the directions that bring them the most joy. The process won't just open them up to all of the possibilities that the world has to offer. If you let it, you'll grow as an adult, and the experience will bring you closer to your children than you ever could have imagined possible.

If we are a collection of our experiences, then we aren't just made up of the experiences that we can easily recall. Although we can't retell each moment of our lives, the feelings that those moments bring are the building blocks that determine who we are, what we want, and how we are willing to go after it. Your child likely won't remember his or her fifth birthday party, but each passing day readies us for the next. If today is boring, sad, and wasteful, then it is likely that those are the qualities of tomorrow that will impact you the most. It's up to you with which aspects of life your child will identify.

We are lucky enough to live within a reasonable distance from the Philadelphia Zoo, and we took Cole there a number of times in the first couple of years of his life. One thing that I noticed about most of the other families was that they would run through the zoo like they were in a race. This practice of racing through hours in the day is one that I've witnessed over the years in all walks of life, and it makes me sad. If you were going to the trouble of packing up your car, driving to the zoo, and paying to get in, why the hell would you not look at the animals? I mean it doesn't make sense; you're there and you paid. If you aren't going to really look around, then you might as well have stayed home and saved the money. For our family, taking our time and immersing ourselves in whatever we did was the way to go.

Have you ever watched a lion eat? I have, but more importantly, I've watched a two-year-old watch a lion eat for the first time. As an adult, your mind fills in the spaces as you witness an event, but children are living each moment second by second. They are mesmerized by new visual data, and they feel what they are seeing as if their nerve endings were touching what they were witnessing.

One warm winter day, Cole and I packed a lunch and went to the zoo. We made our way into the big cat house and staked out a bit of the old bleacher section that once existed in the building. Careful to arrive before feeding time, we sat down and watched the lions and tigers pace methodically in their cages as they waited for their meal. Cole was wearing a little baseball hat and a Toy Story jacket, I'll never forget. He sat so still and watched the cats as they became more and more fervent in their pacing of the cage. When the keeper brought in the raw meat, the roars from the cats switched from periodic moans to constant, excited growls.

Cole's eyes were wide open, and his head scanned the scene left to right quickly as he took it all in. He watched with awe as the keeper put the food into each cage, and then he picked up his sandwich and ate with the cats. I didn't know where to look. Part of me wanted to only watch Cole's face as he took in all of these new sights, but I was equally interested in watching the animals as they tore at the meat. I realized that while

I had been to the zoo dozens of times in my life, I never really had sat and watched like we were then. I was seeing something new in something that I'd seen before, and I owed it all to Cole. I got to watch those lions through the eyes and soul of a two-year-old boy, through my son.

This is where life happens, where children's sensibilities are formed, and where adults can see the world one more time, like it was the first time. Watching your child watch the world is like learning life from the ground up, but this time with an adult's mind. You'll be surprised at what you see when your parent's perspective and your adult cynicism are stripped away. This is your chance to again see the pure nature of the world, to remember the possibilities that you felt as a youngster.

Get your kids out into the world, and let them see as much of it as you can. Find the stuff that you love, stuff that you hate, and the things you never tried. Let them see it all so that they can figure out what makes them feel passionately. Dangerous elements aside, don't try and control which experiences get to be part of the recipe that creates who they'll be one day. They will gravitate to the things that they feel most strongly about. Interpret that attraction as an indication of what life wants for them.

I've seen children pushed to be doctors, teachers, parents, and straight. When those children grow up, they all end up having two things in common—they have proud parents and live unhappy lives. It will take a grand amount of bravery for you to expose your children to all that the world has to offer. Sit with them as you both see things for the first time. You won't be sure of how they will react, but if it's your goal to raise a happy person then this you must do without judgment, ego, or foregone conclusion of what the future will bring. They'll come to you when they are unsure of their next step, and that's when the parenting happens. Until then, just enjoy watching them live, learn, and grow.

I May Be Growing Ovaries

I made the decision to stop wearing sweatpants one day at lunch. We were in one of those play areas in a fast food restaurant. I was running around like crazy that morning, doing all sorts of errands, when I realized that no one had eaten in quite some time. We stopped at the first place that we saw, grabbed a burger, and descended into the playroom where Cole quickly ate and then ran to climb on the sliding board maze.

I had our mail in my bag. I remembered that one of my favorite magazines was in the pile, so I leaned back in my chair, cracked it open, and picked at the chicken-like food that I bought for myself. I was momentarily as happy as I could ever hope for. My son was safe and busy, and no one needed me. On the beach in St. John couldn't have felt any better at that moment.

A few minutes later, a kid came flying out of the sliding board chute, screaming his head off. His shrill cry pulled my face out of my magazine, and I made eye contact with a mother across the room. We both smiled that smile that says, "I knew that wasn't my kid." When she looked away, my eyes stayed on her. She looked ragged. She was pretty, but she came off as if someone had forgotten to tell her that she was. Her hair was a wreck, her face looked soft, the bags under her eyes were dark, and the light was gone from her eyes. She was dressed like she planned on spending the day in bed with the flu—nasty sweatshirt, a quickly thrown together ponytail, and a pair of sweatpants that screamed "I've given up." The sight of her made me wonder about the rest of the people in the room, so I began to scope out the other moms. Two facts quickly jumped out at me— I was the only man in a room full of about twenty adults, and everyone was wearing sweatpants, even me.

This was the first time that I can remember thinking that I was living what would generally be accepted as my mother's life. I began to notice that I was never around men, that everywhere I went it was just the girls and me. Every back-to-school night consists of the teacher, me, twenty ladies, and two fathers who couldn't think fast enough on their feet to get out of coming along with their wives.

When we were designing our home, the architect was furiously taking notes about the things that we hoped to be able to afford to build. Kelly gave her list, and then he turned to me. I said, "I'd like the laundry room to be on the second floor." I couldn't think of anything better than eliminating standing in the dank, dusty basement from my life. Much of what I do, say, and feel is directly connected to my being a full-time, stay-at-home dad.

My wife has been asked at our son's baseball games how she gets Cole's pants so white. She just smiles and points to me. It always feels like other people expect me to be embarrassed, but I couldn't be further from embarrassed, I'm proud. I can tell the difference between my son's socks and mine when I sort the laundry, without taking my eyes off of the ball game. My system for rotating food in the cabinets is unmatched. I move cups onto coasters, turn off the lights that everyone else leaves on, and adjust the thermostat before bed to save us a few dollars. I know the best times of day to grocery shop without crowds, manage our children's social calendars, take them to their games and practices, and bug them to blow their noses. All proudly.

After helping another mom out with something that I think she believed to be a female-only task, she looked at me and asked how I knew what to do. I raised my hand to my eye, while holding my thumb and forefinger very close to each other, and answered, "I'm this close to growing my own set of ovaries."

Back to the sweatpants … I've never worn them in public again because I associate them with giving up. I left that fast food restaurant determined to not become one of those ladies. However, in the years that have followed, I've learned that my evaluation of those women was unfair and shallow. I wish that I could find them all so that I could apologize.

In the years since then I've learned that mothers are the key to everything. I've lived my life with them for well over a decade, and it cannot be stated firmly enough that the planet isn't referred to as "Father Earth" for a reason. Much like the place that we all call home, our mothers are the center that keeps all of our collective feet from floating into space. Mothers are all things to all children, and each of us is someone's child. It's the most important job in the world, and I feel blessed that I have been able to do it. I would, count anyone foolish who undervalues the endless giving that emanates from a mother. Being a stay-at-home dad makes me want to call my mom and thank her every day. Having the privilege of watching our children perpetually change, learn, grow, and adapt makes me want to hug Kelly and not let go. I am as grateful for this opportunity as I am saddened that my having it means that she can't.

I saw a movie back in 1996 called *Microcosmos*. It's a documentary about insects. The filmmaker used incredible close-ups and time-lapse photography that gave me as the viewer the feeling that I was standing next to some of the most amazingly varied and fascinating living things on the planet. Slowing down the filming let me examine each step of each frame in a way that left me feeling like I'd experienced the subject's entire life in just a few moments. As truly awe-inspiring as the film was, my real takeaway leaving the theater was the knowledge that all of this was going on all around me and I never knew it.

It may sound a bit crazy, but that is how I see motherhood. Each day is full of wondrous and critically important moments. Endless decisions are made and carried out by our moms in homes all around the world. Each step holds the hope of survival, growth, and prosperity, but as important and plentiful as these women and their work are, it goes unseen by most. When someone does finally pay attention, it's unlikely that the viewer will take the time to learn about the complexities of these seemingly simple tasks. You can watch bees collect nectar and dismiss it as just bugs eating, or you can spend a few minutes understanding how their repetitive act literally makes the world spin.

This chapter is dedicated to the women I know who asked me if my book was going to help their husbands to understand what they do all day. I hope this is what you had in mind, girls. I don't just think that you are the center of everything, I know that you are. I may not be a woman, but I try very hard to be even half the mom that I know my gorgeous wife would have been if our lives would have gone a different way. I hope every day that I am making Kelly proud, while properly representing all that you ladies do, feel, and love so diligently when no one is looking.

Baseball, Part I

My father never let his guard down. Until he left our home, he was forever acting the way that he thought a father and husband should act. We rarely ever got to see him be himself, but late one night in October of 1980, because of baseball, I got to see my dad be the guy he was before I knew him. The second after Philadelphia Phillies' pitcher Tug McGraw threw his hands in the air to signal their World Series victory, my dad leapt from our sofa not knowing which way to run first. He initially flew out onto our patio and just screamed, but that didn't seem to satisfy whatever urge he was feeling, so he sprinted to the kitchen and then ran out of our front door holding some of our pots and pans.

I was only nine years old, and I didn't know what was happening. I made my way outside to find out where he went and why he took our pots, but before I could get to the door I heard the strangest noise. I would learn in a moment that the sound I'd heard was made by countless people banging pots and pans together. When I got outside, I looked to my left and there was my father, as joyous as I'd ever seen him, or as it turns out, would ever see him again ... letting out his jubilation through our cookware.

Twenty-three years later, I saw our three-year-old son Cole swing a baseball bat for the first time. It wasn't a real bat, but rather one of those fat hollow plastic ones that you can buy in a toy store, the ones that come complete with an equally oversized tee and plastic balls. One spring day Kelly and I took Cole into our backyard to see if baseball might be a good activity for him. We set up the plastic tee and showed him how to swing his new bat, and then we stepped back to let him explore. Cole immediately stood next to the tee in exactly the correct position, as if he'd done it a million times before. His hands moved slightly back, his front foot lifted ever so gently from the ground; as he strode forward his hands moved quickly, and when the fat bat hit the plastic ball, it flew forty feet straight ahead and in a perfect line. Kelly and I looked at each other in a moment of amazement, and then we put the next ball on the tee to find out if what just happened was a fluke or foreshadowing. Cole hit those balls again and again that afternoon, each time straight ahead and farther than we expected that a small boy with a plastic bat could.

It's now ten years later, and Cole still gets off of his bus, no matter the time of year, and asks me if I have time to go outside to have a catch with him. He asks on cold days, hot days, rainy days, and days when he doesn't feel well. At the holidays when we ask him what he would like as a gift, he always responds first by saying, "I could use a new bucket of balls." He loves playing baseball in a way that I never imagined was possible, and his enthusiasm has strengthened mine to the point where I can say that watching him play is one of my life's great joys.

If you aren't a baseball person, you may not be aware of the sound that a crisply thrown ball makes when it hits the pocket of a glove just right. It's a sorta "thwap" sound that erupts quickly, and when it happens just right, you know that it stung the hand of the person catching the ball. Once you've heard this surprisingly loud and distinctly unique sound, you'll never mistake it for anything else. When two people are having a catch with a baseball the back and forth settles into a rhythm that's marked with a "Thwap, <pause>, thwap, <pause>." As the throwing begins to intensify, the ball moves faster and faster, and when it reaches a certain speed you can hear it cut through the air: "Ssss, thwap, <pause>, ssss, thwap, <pause>." These simple noises and the pauses in between make up perhaps my favorite sound in the world. They cause me to think of my son every time I hear them, no matter who is throwing and catching the ball.

When I sit in the bleachers to watch Cole warm up with one of his teammates before a practice or game, a peaceful calm falls over me. There is something so very beautiful about watching him play this game, a game that he loves so much. When his experience is combined with mine and it plays out in front of me with the melodic rhythm of the thrown ball as its score, I feel perfectly centered inside.

There is only one thing that bests watching Cole learn, enjoy, and excel at baseball—standing together with him in our backyard and having a catch. When we throw together I often have to resist the urge to run across the grass and hug him. Instead we use the time to talk about his day, he asks about mine, we talk about great plays that we saw in the majors the night before, sports news, school, whatever. He loves to try to trip me up with the stupid jokes that he and his friends tell one another at school. I ask if the girl he likes is still around, and he looks sheepishly at the ground when he answers. It's the perfect time to say all of the things that we want to say to each other; it's our father-son time.

Sometimes we throw in silence; other times he helps me with my grip, and he loves to show me that his arm is getting stronger than mine. We'll joke with each other, bust balls a bit, and then go back inside the house so I can make dinner. It's the best part of my day with him, and if he enjoys it even slightly as much as I do, then I know he's having a great time, too. I realize that one day he'll move out of our house and we won't have this time together anymore, but I feel comforted in knowing that wherever he is, no matter how far away or how long since I've seen him last, I'll be able to turn on a baseball game and hear the sounds that will bring me right back to this perfect moment in my life.

Baseball, Part II

Baseball gives many fathers and sons the ability to connect, but it also provides the opportunity to draw parallels to which your son can relate. I often find myself talking with Cole about life in baseball terms, and I think that for him it makes hearing the lessons that he needs more relatable and easy to absorb.

Recently Cole hit his first batting practice home runs during an all-star tryout. He has played on our town's all-star team with the same great bunch of boys for years. Every summer for six or so weeks those boys eat, sleep, and live baseball together. They practice nearly every day to play in a local tournament that, if won, will lead them to a regional, which could lead to a state and beyond. It's all part of the Little League Baseball system and is taken quite seriously in youth baseball circles. Prior to this tournament in the late spring, there is a tryout for a team such as this in almost every town across the country. I'm proud to say that Cole has been an all-star every year since he was seven years old.

Cole has come very close in a number of games this spring to hitting a home run, but it wasn't in a game that he hit his first few—it was in batting practice during his all-star tryout. There is a big difference between hitting a ball off a pitcher in a game and hitting one from a coach who is throwing the ball right down the plate to you. Nevertheless, this was the first time that Cole was able to move the ball through the air with enough proficiency that it cleared the two-hundred-foot fence. I was excited for him, not because these were home runs, because technically they were not, but excited because he reached another goal that he set for himself. He hit a ball over the fence on the field that he's played on for most of his life. Not really a home run, but a memory he doesn't want to forget for sure.

It's rather customary for children to keep the home run balls that they hit over the fence. I wasn't sure if Cole would want these particular balls because they weren't hit in a game, but I retrieved them just in case. I passed Cole as I walked back to where Kelly and I were sitting; he was now on the field playing his position. I spoke to him through the fence and asked, "Do you want to keep these?" He turned his head just so slightly and grinned ever so slimly so as not to look too excited in front of his teammates, a few of whom had already hit home runs in actual games. He nodded his head yes, just enough so that I could see, and I smiled back and said, "Do you want just the first one or all three?" He held three fingers at his side without looking back at me. He knew that the boys were going to give him crap for keeping those balls, but he wanted them anyway. With that I was now proud of him for something else, for being his own person.

The next day Cole told me that many of the boys on his team gave him some good-natured ribbing about keeping the batting-practice home run balls. They teased him a bit about it and gave him their opinions about the matter, as boys will do. Cole just laughed along with them knowing that they really didn't care, they were just doing what friends do, acting like boys and busting balls just like he and I do sometimes when we throw. He loves being a part of that club and didn't seem in any way put off by the hazing that he was receiving.

Still, as his father, it's my job to ensure that my child is experiencing this banter in a healthy way. The next time we were alone, I brought up the subject so we could talk about it. Not unexpectedly, when I told him I was proud, he minimized the accomplishment. Instead of disagreeing, I gave him the respect that his feelings deserved and told him that I understood that he didn't feel like they were real home runs. We spoke about goals and surpassing and setting new ones. He agreed that now that he knew he could clear the fence his new goal was to do it in a game. I nodded to indicate that I thought he was right, and then gently asked what the boys on the team said to him about his keeping the balls after the tryout.

He told me what each had said and that he knew they meant it a little but that he believed at the same time that they were just messing with him in a friendly kind of way. I was happy that he wasn't being oversensitive, and

I told him again how proud I was of him for not buckling to peer pressure. I smiled to myself knowing that he was well on his way to being his own man.

Then, I told him the story about that big plastic bat when he was three. He'd heard it before, but this time I told the story from my perspective instead of from his, letting him know how my heart sees our life together. When I finished telling Cole how excited Kelly and I were when he found a sport that he'd love on that day so long ago, he asked why, and I told him, "Because we love you so much and we want you to have every great experience that you can." He liked that answer, and then we both became a little quiet.

Cole broke the silence by saying that he still felt weird for taking the balls home after he hit them out during batting practice. "Maybe," I said, "maybe one day if you have children, you'll get to take your son into your backyard and have a catch with him. You could take one those balls out of a drawer and make your own memory with your boy. Tell him how this ball was the first one his daddy ever hit over a fence, explain to him about setting goals, and the hard work and the perseverance that it takes to reach them. Be sure to tell him how you felt when you reached your goal and how excited you were to set a new one." I paused, then added, "Maybe you can tell him about us and all of the great times that we had having a catch in the yard you grew up in. Then, use that ball to teach him to love baseball the way you do, and the way I do when you are with me. Tell him that it isn't the game that you love most—not the stories or the heroes, the close games, or the big wins. Show him that this game means more than all of that to the fathers and sons who experience it together and know that, wherever I may be, I'm thinking of you and me and all of the 'thwaps' that we made together."

Those three balls are now displayed in a case on Cole's bedroom wall. They are waiting patiently until it's time to make another little boy feel what only baseball can ... and waiting to help my son learn what it means to be a father.

I Remember Having Sex ... and the Baby Proves It!

It might not surprise you

that I considered other titles for this chapter ... "How I Lost My Gig as My Wife's Boyfriend and Made My Penis Hate Me" or "Having a Baby Taught Me That Condoms Have an Expiration Date" or "Is It Masturbation If My Wife Is in the Room?" You get the point.

I now believe that the first time Kelly felt my son kick inside of her, the process of phasing me out as her number-one guy began. Any chance of continuing on as the most important man in Kelly's life ended abruptly when our son Cole came into the world. Suddenly I wasn't the cutest guy in the house, and I certainly wasn't as interesting as I once was. My best jokes began to fall flat, and my advances were rebuked. It didn't take me long to see the writing on the wall—I wasn't Kelly's boyfriend anymore; Cole was.

It's clear to me that there are stages of a human's life and that we are often powerless to break free of what nature intends for us. When Kelly gave birth to Cole, his arrival unleashed a part of her that I don't think she imagined existed before our baby was born. She almost instantly became a different person; having a baby fundamentally changed who she was. Her perspective shifted, personal goals dissipated, and what she desired from her life began to morph. All Kelly wanted was what was best for our baby. Giving birth is transformational, life affirming, and unlike anything that a person who hasn't lived through the experience can imagine. Man or woman, you will be different after you have a baby.

We went in an instant from being "Kelly and Scott" to being "Cole, Kelly, and Scott." On one hand, I think that it's beautiful how fast love connected us. I absolutely believe that being so enraptured by one's family is one of the great experiences that a person can have in this life. My penis, however, is not a fan of what all of this meant to him.

Kelly became so fixed on Cole that most days I felt like I didn't matter to her anymore. Within six months of his birth, it seemed that my wants, needs, and desires were not incorporated into decisions, and we just stopped being intimate with each other the way we once were. It was as if the birth of our son meant that reproduction had successfully happened and thus I was no longer required.

It was a conflicting time in my life. I was as happy as I could possibly expect to be about my son and the family that Kelly and I created, but, at the same time, I was mourning the exciting and fulfilling relationship that I had had with my best friend. Gone was sitting together for no reason. We stopped playing chess and seeing movies. Everything we did became centered around the baby. I was prepared for our lives to change, but I guess that I didn't expect that we would so completely lose ourselves in the process or that our relationship would change so drastically.

What I didn't recognize at the time is that I was changing also. Kelly wasn't the only one succumbing to the will of Mother Nature. In the exact moment that

Kelly was being transformed into a mom by whatever it is that controls our inner selves, I was turning into a dad. I became rigid and felt as if there were rules to life to which I suddenly had to adhere. In the exact moment it became difficult for Kelly to remember that we were bonded together before we had a baby, I was becoming less likable as a candidate for her affection. In hindsight, I can't say for sure that these factors could have been overcome just then. If I were able to coach a young couple who just had a baby, I doubt that even my best advice could keep them from becoming what nature intended them to become as they accepted responsibility for another life. Maybe that's just how it's supposed to be. Perhaps one of us prevents over-breeding while the other defends the new family against unknown outside dangers.

If you have ever watched a nature show, you know that some male mammals just walk away when the mating process is finished. Others leave after the babies are born, but not many stick around and make what we think of as a family. We humans are arguably more advanced, but it still occurs to me that our chosen path is one that deviates slightly from nature's intent. I'm not saying that fathers should walk away, but I suspect male animals do this so that they can continue to reproduce. Unlike other mammals, I don't have any desire to populate the world, but I definitely was not finished having sex just because we had a baby. No one cares about Mars and Venus, ladies ... it's all about our penises.

Like most misunderstandings, the one between men and women pertaining to sex is clouded further by the fact that we don't speak about it clearly and honestly. Puritanical embarrassment takes over, and we, like children, try to joke our way through the conversations that mean the most to us. Trite comments and tired jokes from men often lead women to believe that all we want is to have sex and that the act for us is mostly devoid of the feeling and depth that is so essential to them. That's only partially true.

What I see most in my own life and from other men is that we often feel beaten. There are only so many times that your ego can withstand being rejected. When I make sexual overtures and my advances are declined, I feel rejected. There is no better way to put it. Intellectually, I may know that Kelly is tired, stressed, and probably more than a bit bored with my outdated moves. However, what she may not know is that she's my girl, the mother of my children, the only woman that I love with the intensity of passion, and that I want to be close with her for more reasons than simply that it feels good. It's devastating to learn that she doesn't feel the same way at that moment.

Girls, listen, I'm about to give you pearls of wisdom … wisdom from a straight man who is living a life that is almost entirely that of a woman. You are going to get the best relationship advice here that anyone could ever hope to receive. I know that it will seem as if I am suggesting that you forgo your feelings to appease your husband's, but it's so much more than that. If you want a happy life with the man whom you chose to be the father of your children, have sex with him. Do it without making him feel as if you are burdened by the task, make it your idea, be spontaneous. Leave your stress, body-image issues, and the rest of life on the floor next to your bra, and throw your husband a bang that he'll never forget … I promise you that he'll start talking to you again.

There's no denying that most men I know aren't the

best communicators. Men may not do a good job of expressing themselves, but take it from me, they love you. They want to grow old with you. They don't care that you've gained weight, look tired, or that your hair isn't the way you want it. They love you.

You ladies have to remember that most men aren't as in touch with themselves as I may be. If you give up on your relationship, their penises will lead them. Simply put, guys need to have sex. It may sound pathetic to you, but we attach our value, manhood, and pride to our ability to do so. In the end, whether you want to believe it or not, you are in nearly complete control of how fulfilled a man your husband feels he is. Making your husband feel valued is not a complicated job or even a difficult one. It doesn't require much effort, and it will pay you back a millionfold. Stroke your husband's ego— make him feel like the guy he was when you met. He still is, and he kicks himself every second that he can't prove it to you. You're the same girl as well, and I think you'll be surprised at how alive you'll feel again when the two of you reconnect.

Could I See You in the Basement for a Minute?

Cole had just turned three years old when Kelly and I began talking about having a second child. I'm sure that Kelly brought up the subject first, but I was more than excited to talk about the possibility. So far, Cole had been the happiest, easiest baby and most pleasant toddler for whom we could have hoped. After his bout with projectile vomiting ended several months in, he never had a medical issue again. (Well, except for the time that we ended up in the emergency room with a knife wound to his toe, but that's neither here nor there. Who knows which one of us left that sharp knife on the floor as we carved Halloween pumpkins? Could have been me; could have been Kelly;

there's no way to know, so let's not dwell on things we can't be sure of [it was me].) Anyway, he was a healthy, happy, fun baby, and we felt ready to do it again.

In the beginning of our talks, we kept the topic pretty informal and surface level. Kelly had one goal for her next conception—to give birth in the summer so that our next child wouldn't always be stuck having indoor birthday parties. My main concern was coordinating our second child's learning to walk with Cole starting school. In my heart I felt like a really good stay-at-home dad, but I still wondered nervously from time to time if my success didn't perhaps have more to do with how easy Cole was as opposed to my considerable skills. The last thing I wanted was an unruly baby walking around and a little boy to parent at the same time. Like having the laundry room on the second floor, at that point it seemed to be of the utmost importance. In the end, I could see the love in Kelly's eyes that she was yearning to give to another baby and I agreed that it was time for one more.

After launching "operation have a baby," the next couple of conversations that we had weren't quite as much fun as the first. We talked about money a lot during these unpleasant conversations. I say unpleasant because the decision to have a baby seems like it should be accompanied by talk of baby names, bedroom colors, and parties. In reality, those things are far sweeter if you don't have a lot of nagging questions about finances in the back of your mind. We wanted to get all of our ducks in a row this time around so that we could really enjoy the process. Everything moved so quickly during the first pregnancy that it felt like we were too busy managing our lives to really live them. This time was going to be different.

After we sat down and proved to ourselves that the addition of another child wouldn't outpace Kelly's growth at her job, we laid to rest the idea that we might not be able to afford to expand our family. We felt that we had enough space for at least the first few years in our current home, so that wasn't an immediate concern.

The tensest conversations were about health. We spoke about in-utero health testing and how we would want to address potential life-changing issues should they arise. Kelly and I both had strongly held beliefs, and they were diametrically opposed. We spoke at length about each of our beliefs, and in the end, Kelly was not willing to bend her convictions to meet mine. Even though I disagreed, I respected how she felt, and I believed that she should have final say in any issues pertaining to her body and the babies inside of it. I withdrew my concern and, thankfully, we never had to revisit either side of the argument while Kelly was pregnant.

With all of our concerns voiced and discussed, there was nothing left to do but wait for October to arrive so that we could get with the baby making. Our best first grade math told us that an October conception gave us the chance to have a baby in May or June.

Married sex is a funny thing. Actually, if I knew for sure that this passage was only going to be read by married people, I could just stop writing after saying that. However, just in case … Married sex is a funny thing is a statement that speaks volumes if you're married. If you're single, that comment will make you feel empathy for all of the sad married people who you imagine do it wrong. I bet you single people think that we don't keep it fresh or try new things, such as role-playing. In reality, we role-play each time we have sex. Here's a sample of my last sexual encounter with my wife to prove it.

Kelly: Leave me alone.

Scott: Come on, please.

K: <Almost inaudible sound of annoyance> Fine.

S: <Smile>

K: Go close the door and lock it.

S: I'm so excited!

K: Idiot.

S: Don't call me an idiot because I'm excited to have sex.

K: Your elbow is on my nipple.

S: Sorry.

Minutes pass...

K: This isn't bad.

S: Thanks!

What you just read was our role-playing. I play the part of an undersexed husband and Kelly is the wife who is years past being excited by my tired moves. Our back-story is fascinating; we are exhausted, nearly broke, and mentally drained by years of caring for the world that we built. End scene.

This next sample is of a sexual encounter before we were married and had kids.

Kelly: Tonight I want to *&^&%#$ 5&*&^%$ #^&^ (&^.

Scott: Um yes, we can definitely do that!

K: I was thinking we could do it outside in a field.

S: Yeah, let's do it outside in a field.

K: Don't forget when you &^%$ my (*&^%^&* I don't like it if the *&^%&* is too *&&**&.

S: Noted.

Fast forward to the field...

K: I wonder if the people on that train could see my &%$#^&*?

S: I don't care ... I love you!

K: I LOVE YOU! Now take your *&^^%& *^%& (&^%^* and *&^%%^&*. I feel sorry for all of the married people that can't keep their sex lives hot!

S: Me too...

Anyway, married sex is funny in that it doesn't often continue in the direction that it set out on when you were dating. Eventually you run out of new experiences to have, and a pattern begins to form. That pattern becomes tired, and what you are left with is married sex.

However, there are a few exceptions to this rule, and one of them is when you try to get pregnant again. When you're trying to have another baby, everything is new again, exciting. Your world feels full of possibilities. Don't get me wrong, the sexual frenzy will stop immediately after conception, and nine months later you'll discover a previously unimagined level of exhaustion, but for the time being, life is very good!

But on with my story ... the week before Halloween in 2003, I was getting laid like twice a day, and it was fantastic! Some sessions were loving, some were down and dirty. We had sex in the living room, on the floor, and even in our bed. Honestly, we did it anywhere we were when it was time to try again. Life was perfect. We were having a lot of fun being together, and the excitement and love in the air was genuinely wonderful. I felt like I was twenty-two again, and Kelly looked as beautiful as I could ever recall. You couldn't wipe the smiles from our faces.

On the evening of Halloween as we were preparing to take Cole out to trick-or-treat, Kelly walked up to me and said, "Can I see you in the basement for a minute?"

My mother had stopped by to see Cole in his costume, so we asked her if she could hang out with him for a few minutes while we talked in the basement. I bet you know what happened when I got downstairs. Kelly didn't want to talk at all. (Brief side note: I can't recommend enough having sex on a denim couch. It's like making love in your jeans without that confined feeling.) I'll never forget the sequence of events that led to Arden's conception. It went like this:

Kelly: (from downstairs) Lock the door.

Scott: Oh, we aren't talking, are we?

K: (On her back, jeans around one leg.) Nope ...

S: <Smile> (I smile a lot when I see Kelly naked.) My mom is upstairs.

K: Then you better be quick.

Don't be jealous, ladies, but I was quick, and accurate, apparently, because Kelly was buying a pregnancy test only days later. In one minute (well, maybe it was three or four), Kelly and I created a person who is today lying on the sofa with our dog as I write this. (Don't worry, it's a new sofa.) I just looked at her and she smiled. I'm going to try and take a picture without her seeing me. I'll be right back. (Took the picture.)

As we planned for the birth, Kelly was adamant that Cole be the first person to hold Arden, so he would come with us to the hospital when Kelly went into labor. It was around midnight the night before Kelly was scheduled to check into the hospital to be induced. Cole had been a full two weeks late, and Kelly's OB didn't want her to go through that again. We were too excited to go to sleep that night, so we were up late packing and taking the last pictures of Kelly pregnant while we could. Kelly is an exceptional beauty normally, but when she is pregnant, she's that much more amazing. I remember being in the kitchen after we took the pictures, when Kelly calmly spoke my name.

"Scott, I think my water just broke," she called.

Based on our experience with Cole, we never really prepared for the idea that childbirth would begin naturally on time. This boneheaded oversight was the first of only a few times that we made the rookie parenting mistake of treating our children as if they were the same person. We packed up the car and woke up little Cole. I was way too excited, and Kelly had to ask me to slow down a few times on the drive to the hospital, even though birth was still a ways off.

One of my favorite moments of the night happened as we walked from the parking garage to the hospital. Cole was too tired to walk, so I sat him on top of Kelly's luggage like a carry-on bag. His butt was on the top of the bag, and he lay back on the extended handle. When I tipped the bag toward me to walk, he was perfectly reclined and holding the huge sign he made that read, "Happy Birthday, Arden!"

Arden arrived on schedule on that morning in July 2004, and she was perfect. Cute little face, light hair, big full lips right for kissing, just like we imagined. This time around was different. Gone was the feeling that I couldn't care for a baby. Past was the idea that any small mistake would result in something horrible occurring. This was my time; I was going to cut a swath through parenting that would make the Sesame Street crew look like they never met a kid. Of course, whenever you plan, life throws you some curveballs.

Sleep— Get It Now

During any pregnancy, there are a number of things that people tell you to be on the lookout for. Most of the advice you'll get will seem obvious. I imagine that you, like me, will take it all with a grain of salt. The only piece of advice that I wish that I had taken more to heart was "Get some sleep now."

Actually that advice is slightly misworded, though I recounted it just as others will say it to you. It's misleading because you can't bank sleep. You sleep when you're tired and wake refreshed. It's not as if I could sleep today away and then stay up for the next three days, using the hours that I got today to keep me going. Sleep just doesn't work like that. If it did, there might be no other walk of life that would benefit more than parenting.

Since Cole was born, I've experienced all of the levels that exhaustion has to offer. My journey began on the first day that he arrived, and if I'm being honest, I'm a bit bleary-eyed right now. From passing out in Kelly's hospital bed on parenting day one to last night's combination of lawn irrigation and blood glucose management, I definitely understand what it is to walk around feeling just a little dopey from lack of uninterrupted sleep.

In May of 2000, when the Philadelphia Flyers and the Pittsburgh Penguins played one of the longest games in NHL history that went into the early morning hours, I was able to see most of it. How, you ask? During his first few months of life, Cole needed a bottle about every two hours. On the night in question, I put Cole down at around ten. I was able to get him to fall to sleep with my patented singing of "Blackbird" by the Beatles, and then I laid him ever so carefully in his crib. I thought for a moment about trying to stay up and watch the end of the Flyers game, but I was just too tired. I knew that if I tried hard, I could get two hours of sleep before Cole got hungry and woke up. Almost exactly two hours later, he woke up hungry. I went back to the living room and turned on the television while I was feeding him, something that I would do when I needed help staying awake during his feedings. Do you know what I saw when I turned on the television? The hockey game that should have been over long ago, now in overtime, still being played. I enjoyed the game for as long as it took Cole to finish, then I changed his diaper, got him back to sleep, and climbed into our bed one more time. The last thing I expected when Cole woke up again sometime after two in the morning was to see that hockey game still going! I realized at that moment that I had something in common with the men skating up and down the ice—we were all exhausted beyond words. Cole and I settled in our chair, and I whispered in his ear that we would stay up this time to find out who won the game. A few minutes later at exactly 2:35 AM, a debilitated Keith Primeau scored for the Flyers. His goal evened the series at two games apiece and left me with a memory of a seemingly innocuous moment with my son that I don't imagine I'll ever forget.

My learning curve for existing on little sleep was a steep one; it took months of long nights with Cole to teach me how to function without it. In the beginning, I wasn't the Zen-like nightwalker that I am now. Back then, I'd wake up on the sofa with a bottle leaning on my face, holding a passed-out baby tucked under my arm. Once I closed my eyes at a red light, just for a second, only to open them again unsure of how long they were closed. These things would have scared me if I hadn't already known that I was a super ninja in my sleep, that my body was in full "protect Cole mode," even when my eyes couldn't stay open any longer.

Kelly rode the train to her job every day for the first eleven years that we were married. Each morning, in an effort to save the parking fee at the train station, I would drop her off at the platform. This was a difficult task for me at times, but one that I enjoyed even though Kelly isn't much of a morning person. I really loved the few minutes that we got to spend together as we made our way through town and to the station. Moreover, I'm a bit of a cheapskate when it comes to spending money on stuff like this, so the savings motivated me a lot on the mornings that I found getting out the door difficult. The worst part was dressing the baby and loading him into that seat without causing too much of a stir. Most days the ride to and from the train would wake me up and get me ready for the day. However on the day that I discovered my true ninja self, I just could not wake up. I felt like I wanted to simply rest my head on the steering wheel as I drove to the train station, and on the ride back, I began explaining to Cole, as if he understood me, that when we got home we were going back to bed.

I was desperate to close my eyes by the time we got back in the house. They were dry and scratchy, like someone had thrown fine gravel in them. I was woozy and my pillow was calling my name. Cole, on the other hand, was wide awake and looking at me with his big brown eyes, ready for the day. I tried putting him in his crib, but he wasn't having any of that. I thought a bottle might make him sleepy, but he wasn't drinking. Cole was very young at this point, only months old, but he was just beginning to roll over on his own. When I finally climbed into my bed, I created a wall of pillows and blankets on Kelly's side of the bed, which was meant to contain him long enough for me to take a ten-minute nap. I settled in, put Cole next to me, and wedged him in between the pillows and my shoulder. As soon as my head hit the pillow, I was gone. I can't be sure if what happened next was a minute after I closed my eyes or an hour, but somehow I turned into a super ninja and saved Cole from the stupidity that my exhaustion caused.

I remember being woken by the terrible feeling that Cole had fallen out of bed. It was then that my ninja-like powers were first thrust into being. My left hand involuntarily flung itself over my body and past the mattress edge. Suddenly, I was clinging to a fist full of Cole's onesie, and my heart was pumping like it was going to burst through my chest. I had caught Cole as he was falling to the floor, but caught him how? I was sleeping. Panicked, but grateful, I slowly pulled my hand up the side of the bed to reveal a very happy and smiling Cole, my hand closed around him like a bear trap. To this day, I don't have any explanation of how my subconscious pulled that off, but I am glad that I didn't let Cole fall from bed. Needless to say, the experience woke me, and we were able to begin our day. That was the first and last time I ever tried to sneak a few extra winks when Cole was awake.

The best part about having a baby is that almost each new day brings a new experience. However, many of the problems that you fight through have finite lives. Lack of sleep, for example, doesn't last forever ... it just seems like it will at the time. Eventually your baby will sleep through the night, and you'll be able to rest up and begin to feel like yourself again.

Of course, that is just about the time you decide to have another baby ...

Platitudes

What happens in the split second between thinking and speaking that so often causes us to communicate with each other in oversimplified words and phrases? Is it discomfort associated with emotion? Do we fear rejection? Or, are the thoughts and feelings that we have just too complicated to put into words?

I was taking a moment for myself in the living room when I first took notice of what was about to rule my day and change the words and feelings I'd share with my loved ones. Kelly was working from home, and, because of the open nature of our floor plan, I was able to see her as she toiled. Throughout the day, I saw aspects of her work life that I never knew existed. She was full of stress and overrun with tasks. People called and emailed every few minutes with problems and questions. She was never able to establish a rhythm or get to the heart of the things that she needed to accomplish that day.

At first, I was merely stunned by the enormity of the life that she leads when we don't see her. But as the day went on, the sight of Kelly at work caused me to feel immense pride, anger, love, and sorrow. I was experiencing the strangest mixture of conflicting emotions. I wanted to save, thank, and hug Kelly all at once. I couldn't separate the notion that we should sell everything that we owned and move someplace where life was simpler from the urge to stand up and shout, "Look at you kicking life's ass and taking names!" That afternoon while I cleaned the dishes and made the beds, I thought about each of those feelings, one at a time.

The strongest of my emotions were anger and pride. I was angry at the world for being the way that it is and causing us to have to put so much effort and time into surviving. Why did Kelly have to work so many hours, put that much of her mental and physical effort into a job? I was angry because this cycle we live in is robbing her of our life, and robbing our family of having her in it as much as we should.

When Kelly ends her day understandably exhausted without the time or energy to focus on herself or interact with her family in the way that she wants, that day has been traded. Traded for food, housing, medical insurance, and the rest of the things that we need to flourish as a family. The irony, of course, is that all of those things were never on the list of why we wanted a family or what we imagined a family to be.

The vision is nearly universal—you'll have a baby and then spend your mornings hanging out in a huge bed with your spouse and new child. Picture you and the person you love most in the world lying warmly under the fluffiest white down comforter that money can buy. Your feet will be entangled with theirs, while the perfect baby that you made together lies between you taking a morning nap. There's just enough sunlight peeking through the curtains that you bought after seeing them on the cover of your favorite magazine to cast the warmest, most beautiful light across your baby's face.

Perfect in every way. Then, as if from your favorite movie, one of you reaches across the baby, takes the other's hand, and says, "I wish we could stay here forever ...," and you do.

In reality, the kids are at school, Kelly is working from home, too tired to put on a bra, and I'm running around like a mad person trying to run our home in silence, while Kelly consistently pushes herself on a daily basis in front of my eyes for gas and mortgage money.

I snap myself back from my magazine-cover-induced dream world and examine the pride that I feel in Kelly. She is and always has been "that person." Hard-working student, dedicated employee, great mom, and my best friend. She busts her ass to make sure that we have what we need, not just to survive, but to flourish. That's love. If the kids and I weren't here, I think she might sit on the sofa, turn on the television, and wait for the house to be repossessed out from under her. I bet she'd walk out the door on the day that the sheriff came with a smile on her face, too. That's how tired she is, but somehow she never stops. Her commute is ungodly, her work intense, the stress is monumental, but she keeps going. Our household needs, family requirements, and the love she gives to our family are astounding.

I stood in our bedroom folding laundry and thinking about all of those things. I was overwhelmed with gratitude and love, and all I wanted to do was tell Kelly everything that I just told you. I gathered my thoughts and walked with a lightness in my heart to Kelly's desk. I was determined to let her feel everything that I felt so that, if nothing else, she would know just how much I loved and respected her sacrifice, determination, and love of our family.

When I reached her, she was on the phone having another mind-numbing conversation about office life. I stood off to the side as the call went on a few more moments. Finally, she looked at me as she disconnected the phone, but her face had so much tension in it that it shocked me. She said, "What?" It wasn't an angry "what," but I could see the seriousness on her face.

I opened my mouth, but the words just wouldn't come out. She looked at me like she wanted to scream, not at me, just scream into the air. Then I did what we all do far too often, what I've been striving to not do since that moment. I oversimplified my thoughts, removed the depth of my contemplation, and stammered as if I didn't quite remember what I had originally approached her to say. "You're doing a great job ... just wanted to see if you needed a drink or something."

As I spoke the words, I was screaming at myself in my mind, "Tell her how brave ... you see her level of commitment to your family ... proud, generous ... say something!" But in the end, I just got her a fresh drink with ice and went on my way.

I may have walked away feeling like an ass, but I was an ass who learned a valuable lesson. I don't speak to the people I love anymore in platitudes. I don't allow myself to be lazy when I communicate. I don't wait for a better time. I stopped letting how I feel exist only in my head. Since this moment I communicate better, and it's making a positive difference in my life. My only regret is that it took me so long to figure it all out.

Clarity, intent, context, delivery. Whether you are speaking about feelings, direction, or love, what you mean is meaningless if the person that you are communicating with misinterprets it. If my body language says one thing while my words say another, you can be guaranteed that my message will fall on deaf ears. When your heart says so much, but your words so little, the depth of your message likely won't be felt.

The people in your life are only able to absorb what they see, and it's up to us to present ourselves clearly so that there can be no misunderstandings. If you are unwilling, unable, or unaware in this arena, eventually your relationship will suffer.

Now, no matter what, I say what's in my heart. If Kelly looks great one evening, I tell her so, but I'm not content to just say, "You look great." If her eyes are particularly fetching, I say just that. If the sight of her moving through our bedroom reminds me of when we were dating or makes me relive what I felt as she approached me at the altar … well, then she should know in just those words.

The same goes for my children. I don't just say, "Daddy loves you." I stop in their room and sit with them. We put down the cell phones and pause the television. I talk to them for a few minutes about my pride in them and how deeply or why I love them. I want my kids to know that they are exactly how I envisioned them, even before I met their mom. They should feel that I always wanted them, and that they turned out so amazingly that even I can't believe it.

In the days and years to come, whether Kelly is at work or the kids have left for college, if I'm dead or alive, my family shouldn't just remember that I loved them because I said so. I want them to feel, to really know in my voice that there is no truer statement in their lives. Not just that "I love you," but why and how. I want them to be able to hear my phrasing, for my voice to meld into the fabric of who they are, becoming indistinguishable from the countless other lessons, words, and influences that they will absorb along their journey.

When the days come that they find themselves sitting quietly and reflecting on our time together, I want the feeling to endure more than the words themselves. Like the difference between being told that you are loved and the feeling of being hugged by a person who loves you. I want them to feel my hug wrapping around them … always.

There's No Such Thing as Gender Specific

When I first became a stay-at-home dad, I thought about certain tasks that I was performing in very gender-specific ways. Eventually my new life helped me to understand that there is no such thing as a woman's or man's task when it comes to raising family—only parental responsibilities.

This topic reminds me very much of an old anecdote about pot roast that I've heard and told over the years. I can't remember where I first heard it, but it makes the point that you should question what you know. The story goes that while preparing dinner one evening, a mother cuts the ends off of a pot roast she is about to put in the oven. Her daughter sees the cuts made and asks the mother why she removes the ends of the roast. The mother thinks for a moment, but doesn't know why she always makes those cuts. She tells her daughter that if she wants to find out she should call her grandmother and ask her, since she is the one who taught her the method. The girl calls her grandmother, but she doesn't know either, responding only that she did so because her mother did. Still not satisfied, the girl contacts her great-grandmother by phone to get the answer for which she is so desperately searching. The woman answers the phone; she is old and weary and has to think for a few minutes before she can recall the answer to the girl's question. Suddenly, the great-grandmother remembers why she cut the ends from all of those pot roasts so many years ago and says, "Oh, that's right, I cut them off because my pan was so short that they didn't fit."

I heard that story when I was young, and it has helped remind me over the years to question things that didn't make sense to me. The more I investigated the standards that I was accepting without thought, the more I found that I was doing a great many things out of habit or sense of propriety. I wasn't bothering to decide what I thought of the world; instead I was happy to just see it through my parents' eyes.

I grew up in a home where my father didn't vacuum, but that doesn't mean that men don't vacuum. It's merely an indication that the circumstances of my father's life didn't lend themselves to this task being taken on by him. It makes sense, right? My father woke up at the crack of dawn every day; he went to work and only returned after the day was done. It would be strange for him to also be responsible for the upkeep of our home. My mother didn't change the oil in our cars or climb the roof if the gutters needed to be cleaned, but she did maintain the aspects of our home life that her schedule and skills allowed for. Of course, the other possibility is that my dad was a sexist ass and wouldn't dream of doing something that he deemed to be "woman's work."

That pot roast story really stuck with me as time passed, and I decided at some point that I was going to start asking "why" a little more. Maybe the things that I believed were rules were really no more than decisions controlled by happenstance, and maybe the people deciding "it" didn't have my sensibility. So, I began to really pay attention, and this is what I saw.

Both men and women are to blame for continuing the idea that there are tasks only done by one or the other. However, if I had to say who was more at fault for this, it would be the guys. There is no doubt that sensibilities have changed drastically since my father walked past our vacuum cleaner guilt-free, but some men still resist doing things that they feel aren't gender specific to them. My mother never went to sporting events with us; she didn't take us to practice or sit in the stands while we played. My mom did her chores and my dad did his, but if my father painted a room, then my mother acted as his support staff, making food and bringing drinks. I never once saw my dad bring my mother an iced tea while she was hanging the laundry to dry, but she surely brought him a drink when he was taking care of his end of their agreement. I don't see my mother's support as negative or subservient; I just think of it as supportive, and I wish that more men had that component to themselves. Most women I know today are more involved with the aspects of parenting that were deemed "father's work" back in my dad's day, and I see them adjusting to these new norms nicely. When men get dragged to the other side of that imaginary gender line, they go kicking and screaming.

Don't get me wrong; men do more today than ever in the past, but they still do it partially under protest. They may not be launching that protest so that their wives can see, but they do put on quite a show when it's just the guys listening. Everything is made out to be a chore. "She wants me to …," "My wife is making me …," "I would but I have to take the kids …"—you get the picture. Unless it's sports related, men bitch when they have to do things that they don't want to do, me included sometimes. We can be like little kids in that regard. The entire show that we put on is wrapped in machismo so that not wanting to help doesn't appear to be rooted in laziness or lack of interest. It's one of the actions that I've witnessed over the years that make me saddest for fathers. You see, the only way to show another guy that you aren't soft, whipped, or taking part in "woman's work" is to malign the parts of family life that fall under that heading. I think that when men do that, they create the sense that being involved in any way with these moments lessens their manhood. And I, of course, believe just the opposite is true.

There is no such thing as gender specific when it comes to being a part of your family. I've seen my children do the most amazing stuff in the craziest places, places that the men I know and their fathers have never been. If you only interact with your family in certain situations and ignore the parts of life that you aren't as interested in, then you will only partially know the people that love you the most.

Kelly and I have been together a long time. We knew each other, then dated, lived together, and finally married, all before the age that most people find a serious relationship. I've known Kelly since she was a girl in her late teens, and she's shared a few stories with me about her childhood. The one that comes to mind right now may seem innocuous, but it carries an important message. Kelly grew up in a home with an older brother and two younger sisters. Kelly loved and excelled at gymnastics, but her sisters were accomplished soccer players. Kelly once told me that her parents would go anywhere and travel great distances to see her sisters play soccer, but her dad hardly ever once saw her perform a gymnastics routine. It didn't matter if she was practicing, competing, or about to win a medal, her dad didn't enjoy gymnastics so he didn't go to see her.

I could tell that this part of her childhood haunted her, and one day I asked her father why he rarely saw her perform. He answered simply, "I don't like gymnastics." He didn't realize then, but he did appear to understand when we spoke about it later, that his condemnation of gymnastics all those years ago hurt Kelly as if he had said that he didn't like her personally. It may be too late for me to explain this in a way that will help Kelly, but I want men to understand that when you say you don't like something that your child so closely identifies with, you are telling that child that you don't like who he or she is.

I'm writing this today only one day removed from taking Arden to a gymnastics class. I have to tell you that there are about a thousand things that I'd rather do than watch gymnastics, but those aren't what I was doing yesterday. It doesn't matter if your children are in a bad play, singing off key in the school chorus, or participating in a sport that you absolutely hate, their activities are for them, and you get to experience their joy, struggle, frustration, accomplishments, and defeats as they participate. I really believe that if you don't witness your children living their lives, it is very difficult to properly help them make their way through that life. Your children's teachable moments can act as teaching moments for you as well.

Sometimes, these moments are so small and, at first glance, may seem insignificant. Maybe it's something as simple as shopping for a dress or being behind them for support as they make a decision about what binder to buy for school. Our children are just that, children. Almost everything they do is new to them, and even when it seems that they've been at it for long enough to not need you, they still like to know that you're there. A lot of these moments happen when you don't expect; they happen in department stores, car rides, and during boring events such as dance recitals.

Men can continue to avoid these moments in life if they want. They can make fun of them behind their wives' backs to save face with their friends. You can be sure that more than a few jokes will be told about the guys who do these things with a willing heart. I just wish that those guys would stop saying, "I don't do that, my wife does," in a tone that's meant to belittle the moment. Peer pressure at this age isn't pretty; it's kind of sad, actually.

Privately most guys wish that they had a closer relationship with their fathers, although publicly they mock those relationships. It just doesn't make sense. Don't you see that you are sending your children down the same path that you privately wish you had never had to walk? Eventually, someone will break the cycle. One of the men in your familial line will put his foot down and say that's enough. Why not let it be you? There are a million great experiences waiting to enrich your life if you can just get the idea out of your head that they aren't for you.

Two
Perfect Years

After Arden was born, I felt confident as a father. Cole was four, going on five, and he was going to spend the next few months getting to know his sister before he would begin kindergarten. It was actually just as Kelly and I had planned. Cole would get to be around Arden all of the time for that first year, and just when she started getting very mobile, he would go off to school.

Arden was different, of course, from Cole as a baby, but she wasn't difficult. In a few months any concerns I had over managing two children dissipated, and I began to feel indestructible again. Cole, Arden, and I were living large during our days together. We went on trips, saw movies, played at the park, and went for walks. Our lives felt like they had fallen out of a movie.

I was always very careful to send Kelly pictures during the day. We'd call her office to let her know what we were up to. If something new happened to the kids, I was always sure to remember the moment in fine detail so I could tell Kelly later. I genuinely thought that connection was important to maintain. I am sure that she appreciated all of our calls, emails, and photos. Actually I know that she loved them. However, I was so busy trying to build a great childhood for our children that I never took the time to wonder what she must have been feeling as our notes arrived in her office.

Kelly, Cole, and Arden left the house today so that I could write in quiet. I need it to be silent when I write. As much as I am enjoying writing this book, I still miss my family when they aren't here. Kelly has been working full-time since we were married, and she has never been able to experience all of the little moments that make being a stay-at-home parent the once-in-a-lifetime joy that it is. It took me a long time, perhaps years too long, to realize the depth of what my wife was missing. Kelly loses moments that will never happen again while she is working, and that unavoidable fact must be sad in a way that I can't imagine. Not just a parent trapped at work, but a mother kept away from her children by the exact responsibility that came with having them.

It doesn't matter if you are a man or a woman staying at home with your kids, you have to be aware that your partner is at work and missing out on some of the most wonderful moments of your children's lives. The knowledge that those moments can't be re-created is crushing at times. In the end, the only answer that I ever could come up with to help Kelly not to feel so isolated while she is at work ended up not being a perfect fix, but I don't think there is an ideal fix. I now take the time to preface my notes with small messages that let her know we are thinking of her. I don't know how much this helps to take away the sting of not being there; it probably doesn't, but at least she knows that we know how much it sucks. My hope is that verbalizing the disappointment can help to, in some small way, to decrease that feeling.

As much compassion as I have for the adults who have children, only to spend a majority of their life working to pay for the family they created, there is another side to the story. Most days at home aren't picture perfect, and the person working often has a very difficult time believing that to be true. In their defense, the elimination of commuting, coupled with the idea that you don't have to shave and get dressed to stay at home, does tend to make the grass look greener, but there is more to our story.

Cole once threw up on me seven times in one day. I had to change both my clothes and his after each explosion. Don't forget that later I was the one who had to launder and put away the clothes. Dirtying my own clothing is disheartening enough, but seeing it sullied by another person when you are the one who does that laundry is pure torture.

I haven't made a decision that affected only me in thirteen years. Most parents believe that they can make that claim, but if you work outside of the home I don't fully accept your assertion. I know (even though you all say otherwise) that there are a few minutes in your car or at work that are just for you. I am a stay-at-home dad. I write and maintain my own web site about being the caregiver of a child with type 1 diabetes. I cut the lawn, do the grocery shopping, cook, and clean. I am trying to start a charity to help children to more easily afford insulin pumps and continuous glucose monitors, plus I am writing this book, and do you know that I just got a text message from my family asking me to do something for them? They know that I'm writing and that my manuscript deadline is in two weeks. The entire reason they are out of the house is so that I can write. It's cool, and I don't mind because I am accustomed to it, but it does make my point. Families see stay-at-home parents as lifelines, and that job is a twenty-four hour commitment. Now if you'll excuse me, I have to order my family movie tickets for tonight … they are too busy shopping for school supplies to order them.

Last gripe, though I could do this all day. This week marks the "I don't know how long" anniversary of my having to ask Cole to pick up his wet towel after a shower. I repeat myself so much that I almost can't stop myself from doing it at this point. This week marks the "I don't know how long" anniversary of my having to ask Cole to pick up his wet towel after a shower.

The other night at dinner I talked to the kids about not making me repeat myself so many times to get them to respond or listen. The irony, of course, is that I've had that conversation with them at least a dozen times this year. This week marks the "I don't know how long" anniversary of my having to ask Cole to pick up his wet towel after a shower. This story might sound familiar to people who work; maybe they repeat themselves to their employees with no hope of a response, too, but you can fire those people or at least talk shit about them with your friends.

Even with that in mind, the beginning of Arden's life was a spectacular but transitional time for us. It was the first time that life didn't feel new at every turn, leaving no time to concentrate on the other important aspects of living life as a family. The parenting lessons took a while to learn, but in the end, they would help me transition from young father to gnarled veteran. I was going to need every bit of the experience that these transition years brought to me when Arden was diagnosed with diabetes.

Life Has a Way of Getting in the Way of Living

Every great moment that I've ever experienced with my family could have been missed. Life really is about the pauses in between the moments. All of the great stuff happens when you least expect it, and it all happens so quickly that you have to know when to, as Ferris Bueller once put it, "stop and look around."

When Cole was three years old he announced that he wanted a doll. I'd be lying if I said that I was initially excited that my son wanted a baby doll, but who am I to decide what he wants? So we went doll shopping. The amount of time that we put into finding the doll he wanted was greater than I anticipated when we left the house that morning. We had to make three trips to different toy stores and meticulously search through hundreds of dolls until he found the one that he wanted. Don't misunderstand; he wasn't looking for something that he saw on television, and this wasn't about a certain brand or style of toy. He was looking for this doll like it was a person whom he had lost. I remember having so much to do that day and feeling like I wanted our search to end quickly and mercifully. However, it was a good thing that I didn't get my wish because the experience ended up showing me that this was one of those moments that I would be forever glad for what I witnessed.

Cole walked into the first toy store with purpose; he strode methodically down the doll aisle and looked each doll up and down like they were in a police lineup. We got to the end of the aisle, and he said, "She's not here." I thought, "She?" I asked him to look again, and then I started to really watch his face as he scanned the dolls. He wasn't misspeaking when he said, "She isn't here." He was looking for something specific. We repeated the process at two more toy stores. The day was beginning to drag on, but I stopped worrying about the time and the things that I wasn't doing because I was getting a real look into Cole's mind. At some point, I actually found myself getting excited to see who "she" was.

When he saw Christina for the first time, he knew it was the doll he was looking for. I can't say enough about that smile on his face, and the payoff that he felt after putting in so much time and effort was pure gratification for us both. Cole kept that doll with him for a long time. He didn't carry it around or pretend to feed her, he just kept it in his room on his bed. It was important to him. I don't know why, but I do know that if I had said no or rushed him around that day, I would never have gotten this look into who he is. I learned that Cole knew what he wanted and wasn't afraid to work to get it, and those are traits that he has held onto as he's gotten older. Cole didn't remember that doll when I asked him about her recently. He also didn't remember pulling her out of a box many years ago and Kelly asking him if he wanted to keep her. I didn't feel any sadness when he said no, because the importance of her time with us didn't have anything to do with the relationship that Cole had with the toy. The doll wasn't the memory—watching Cole search for her that day, that was the memory.

Life is the stuff that has to happen. Going to work, washing the dishes, and paying bills. Living is the reason you do those things. So many times we let life interfere with living. It has to be that way sometimes, of course. You're going to miss some of the stuff, and missing out is going make it feel at times like you've failed to be the parent you wanted to be. If you can find a way to appreciate and absorb the moments that happen while life has your attention, I promise that will more than make up for the stuff you can't be there for. You'll make it to your fair share of those big-ticket moments, but don't miss the stuff that happens in between because you are too busy doing life's chores.

Arden finds something important to tell me every time I climb onto our lawn mower. I want to say something quickly just in case Arden finds herself reading this later in her life. Not once so far have you stopped me from cutting the lawn to tell me something that seemed important or that couldn't have waited. Each time you trot across the lawn with that beautiful smile on your face, Arden, I go right into my routine. I have to stop the blade, make sure that you don't get too close, turn off the motor, and pause my radio show. Then you come closer and smile again, somehow bigger than the moment before, and say my name. It doesn't matter what you want to say or if it's important or urgent, you just want to see me. All you really want is to interact with me while I'm doing this thing that you don't normally get to be involved in. It's exciting for you; it makes you happy, and that's all that matters. I don't concentrate on the fact that my nose is running from the dirt in the air or that it's a hundred degrees and humid when you come flying across the yard. The lawn can wait for the few minutes that it will take me to make my girl's day by doing nothing more than talking to you and letting you feel that you have access to me whenever needed.

Even if I am overthinking this moment and Arden's visits are only about how much she just loves to bug me when I'm busy, who cares? Arden loves it and it makes me forget the pound of dust that I inhaled when I cut the dry part of the lawn down by the street.

What you are really doing for your kids when you don't allow life to get in the way is creating a sense of availability with them. You don't want there to be even the slightest idea that there is any impediment between you and them when they want or need to reach out. I don't care how busy you feel, make the time. My parents would have told me, "We're busy," "I'm making dinner," or "I'll get to it after this is finished." We resisted the urge to do the same, and now our children have a healthy anticipation that Kelly and I are here for them whenever they need us. I can't tell you how many drive-by hugs and kisses I get. Even now that Cole has gotten older and entered the age that I honestly thought would signal an end to this connection, he'll walk up to me and just lean into me. He hugs and doesn't let go for a few moments. Most of the time when I ask him if he's okay or wants to talk he just says, "Love you." If that's not worth an extra fifteen minutes to cut the lawn, then what are we even doing?

Life does get in the way of living, but most everything that life requires of you can wait long enough for you to refocus and kiss your kid. There are always going to be exceptions but guard carefully that those exceptions don't slowly become the rule. You don't want to miss this stuff—these moments are the icing.

Her Breath Smells Funny

In the summer of 2006, our daughter Arden celebrated her second birthday with a huge backyard party. There was cake, tons of friends and family, and a giant water slide. It was a perfect day, sunny and warm, but not too hot. The grass was thick and lush, and I recall not wearing shoes because it felt so good between my toes.

Arden being born in the summer is truly the only decision that Kelly and I have ever planned in advance. We are more of a fly-by-the-seat-of-our-pants couple. Normally, we plan vacations only weeks before leaving and wonder aloud after a baseball practice what to do for dinner. We don't plan anything, ever, but we planned to have Arden in the summer so that she could have parties in our backyard. Big, overblown summertime parties with balloons and water slides, ponies, and whatever else we could dream up.

After the excitement of Arden's second birthday wound down, I began to get our house back in order so that we could go away on a family vacation. We were leaving for the beach in two weeks, and there were bills to pay, arrangements for the mail pickup had to be made, and Arden had to go to her two-year-old well child doctor's visit for inoculations and a physical. When all of my ducks were in a row, I made one final stop at my mother's so we could say goodbye.

It was during that visit at my mom's that I changed Arden's diaper and found something that worried me terribly. Her bowel movement was dry. I don't mean just firm, I mean mummified. I couldn't imagine how she passed it. It scared me into calling our pediatrician, who said that she was probably dehydrated and to give her more liquids. Actually, in hindsight, Arden hadn't been feeling well since her well visit. I was certain at the time that she was just running a bit of a fever, probably from one of the inoculations that she received. With that in mind, I felt good about the doctor's assessment, and we both agreed that she'd likely be feeling better soon. With our trip scheduled for the next day, I trusted my instincts, as wrong as they were, and kept on with the task of getting us packed and ready to go.

We drove for almost four hours to get to the vacation house that Kelly's parents had rented for her entire family. In the third hour of the trip, we stopped to get drinks. Arden had recently transitioned from bottles, so she selected and quickly finished a very large beverage. Her thirst didn't strike me as odd at the time, nothing out of the ordinary. An hour later when we reached the house, I went to the back seat to unbuckle Arden. When I reached down her side to get to the buckle, my hand was submerged in liquid. She didn't drink that entire thing, I thought, she spilled it. I lifted her out of the car and realized that her diaper was filled to its capacity and the liquid was indeed urine. Lots and lots of urine. In the hustle and bustle of arriving at the house and the excitement of being on vacation, I didn't give the moment its proper consideration. Looking back, of course, I can see that something was wrong, but at the time it just all eluded me.

The two days that followed were not fun for Arden or me. She was sick and getting sicker, so we'd stay in the house all day together while Kelly took Cole to the beach with the rest of our family. I tried to take Arden out on the second afternoon, but she just stood in the sand motionless. When I think back on that moment, she was so lifeless, like she was dying. I quickly took her back to the rented house, where she ate voraciously and then passed out in bed for hours upon hours. I was so worried about her but really thought that she was fighting a virus of some sort. At sundown that evening, Kelly and I tried to take Arden to a nearby nature reserve. We walked a bit by the water, stared off into the sunset, and even saw a red fox run by. None of the things around us could break Arden's thousand-yard stare, so we took a few pictures of Arden and the sunset and went back to the house.

Late that night, we all gathered around the large rectangular table in the living room to play a board game. It was nearing midnight, and Arden was sleeping on Kelly's lap. I was at the opposite end of the table. The game was fun. I don't remember what it was called, but we were all having such a great time. During one of the lulls in the game, I got Kelly's attention from across the room and said to her, "I meant to tell you earlier that Arden's breath smelled weird to me today."

Kelly asked, "Weird how?" and I responded, "I don't know ... metallic, maybe sweet ..." I watched Kelly's face as it appeared to slide off of her skull. She looked horrified, and as she opened her mouth to speak, I knew what she was going to say. Everything just clicked for us both in that moment. Then Kelly uttered these words: "Arden has diabetes."

We grabbed a laptop and quickly looked up the signs and symptoms for type 1 diabetes. There were five signs listed on the web site that we found. We were able to confirm from what we had seen in the last few days that Arden had four of them. The last indicator, the only thing left between hoping and knowing, was a high blood glucose value. Determined that our daughter would not have diabetes and powered by the insane feeling that uncertainty brings, I ran to my car and sped around that beach town searching for a twenty-four-hour drugstore.

I was going to buy a glucose meter and prove our theory wrong.

I stayed pretty together as I drove up and down those dark, vacant, unfamiliar streets. It took some time, but I found a police officer and he gave me directions to a pharmacy one town over. My steps were measured as I walked the aisle. I was in a hurry to get back to Arden, but at the same time I didn't want to leave that store. When I returned to the house, we read the directions that came with the meter, readied the equipment, and pricked a hole into Arden's fingertip, causing her to bleed.

Kelly touched the test strip to the blood and the meter beeped a few moments later. The meter flashed its message to us, "HI." We frantically pored over the instruction manual, hoping that "HI" meant something good, because we were expecting a number. As it turned out, glucose meters don't have the ability to register a reading when the number is more than four or five times the average glucose level. This meant Arden's blood glucose level was at least 400, possibly more.

With Kelly still in her bathing suit from earlier in the day and me in a pair of shorts, we left the house with

Arden in search of a hospital. It was one thirty in the morning. We touched the "Emergency" button on our navigation system and began to follow the computerized voice to what would soon be the most painful and sad moment in any of our lives. We got caught at a red light on a deserted road. I probably should have just driven through that light, but instead I turned to Kelly and said what is possibly the most mature and parental thing that I have or perhaps ever will say. "Arden has diabetes. I know you're scared and sad, so am I, but this is one of the moments that we have to be strong for her."

I don't know if I was talking to Kelly, me, or both of us, but what I did know was that no one prepares you for a moment such as this. We all talk about the bullet that we'd be willing to jump in front of for our kids, but few of us ever really have to find out if we actually have the courage to leap when the gun is fired. If we were ever going to fall apart, ever going to fail as parents, I worried that this would be the time. That moment felt like the spot in a movie where one of the actors blurts out the obvious so that the last act of the movie has a certain plot direction. I desperately wanted our story to follow the right path to the credits.

I could tell you in minute detail of every moment that passed after I saw the look on Kelly's face back at that beach house. I know what kind of cars I parked next to at the hospital and the appearance of the building in the distance while we were stopped at that traffic light. I could tell you that the place in the emergency room where they put us was about ten feet wide and fifteen across, with a small desk, a computer, and two chairs for us to sit in. Arden's bed seemed to be normal size, but so much bigger after she was in it. The monitors were on her left, we were on her right, and the first doctor that we saw wasn't the one who delivered the news.

It was sometime around three thirty in the morning when a man we had never met before told my wife and me that our daughter had type 1 diabetes and that "her life would never be the same." I've always been thankful that Arden was sleeping when we heard the news because I couldn't stop crying. I would have been even more devastated if I had cried in front of her. They ushered us into a tiny room outside of the ICU. I hesitate to call it a room, actually, because it was a space with a door, just large enough to hold an ugly vinyl loveseat and a small table with an outdated magazine. The nurse told us that they were going to stabilize Arden's blood glucose and then come and get us. She told us we should rest, but what I think she meant was to get some sleep now because this would be our last opportunity for rest.

Kelly and I sat down, and without saying a word or even making eye contact, we leaned into each other and fell asleep. What I remember clearest about sitting down on that loveseat was that when we leaned on each other I felt something that I had never experienced before in my life. I could feel Kelly's desperation and grief through her skin, and I was sure that she could feel mine. It was like the feeling that you get at a funeral when sadness is all around you and the idea that you can escape it leaves you. A tangible void is created under your sternum, and it feels like it is growing and consuming your stomach and chest. The tips of my fingers felt sad, and I struggled to form a coherent thought. These hours were, and hopefully will remain, the saddest that I've ever experienced in my life. My parents' divorce, fights with Kelly that I thought would break us up, opening my eyes in the moments after being in a car accident, none of it comes close to the mix of sadness, anger, helplessness, and indescribable pain that permeated every cell of my body. If there is something coming in my life that will hurt more than this, I am very thankful that I can't, at this time, imagine what it may be.

I haven't slept through the night since I woke up in that space to the voice of the nurse telling us that we could go see Arden. I don't complain about lack of sleep anymore, and it doesn't overwhelm me. Now I know. Now I have a perspective on life that mercifully few others can claim. It took me some time to adjust, but I don't need more than four, maybe five, hours of sleep a night, and the hours don't have to be consecutive. The only thing that matters is that Arden's blood glucose doesn't drop so low overnight that she dies in her sleep.

The knowledge that Arden was walking around the night before at that nature reserve with a blood glucose value well over six hundred is a lesson that struck at me to my core. Our daughter was literally dying in front of us, and we thought she had a virus. The doctors told us that we should be proud that we figured out that she had diabetes before she lapsed into a coma, which they estimate would have happened in another twenty-four hours or so. I've never been able to feel pride in that, even though they say that many children come through the doors unconscious. I'm glad that didn't happen to Arden, but far too guilty to be proud.

When we walked through the ICU to get to Arden, we passed children that seemed far sicker than a child should be. When the nurse pulled back the curtain, I saw Arden, all nineteen pounds of her, propped up in a bed that could have held her twenty times over. There were so many tubes and wires coming out of her arms and chest. I don't know why, but they made me think about her birthday party that had just happened two weeks earlier, and I couldn't make sense of how we got here. I just thought, "She's only two. Do little kids get sick like this when they're two?" I was sure that the answer was no, but then what were all of those tubes for?

In that moment, as if programmed to do so, Kelly took Arden and held her. Then she asked the nurse to help get Arden into her lap. Mother and daughter sat on the chair next to the hospital bed together. The sight of Kelly holding Arden made me realize that we shouldn't have let them separate us, and I wonder to this day about the hours that we were apart. There was nothing to say or to do—the girls just sat there and I just stared at them. Sometime later Kelly told me that I should go back to the house, check on Cole, and get her something to wear because she was still in her bathing suit. She told me not to rush back too quickly. "Make sure that you spend time with Cole before you come back … and get a shower."

When I returned a few hours later, Kelly was in the exact same position as when I had left her. I asked how she was doing. She said that her legs were asleep and that she had to use the bathroom really bad. I asked her why she didn't go sooner and she told me that she couldn't bear to leave Arden alone. I knew in that moment, beyond a shadow of a doubt, that I had married the most wonderful woman in the world. Kelly would have sat there until the end of time with our daughter if she had had to, and she would have done it without an ounce of regret.

It has been more than six years since that day. It's my job to keep an eye on Arden's glucose levels overnight, as well as during the day. There are times that I don't go to sleep until three in the morning. Some nights are steady and easier, but others require multiple blood glucose checks at intervals that make sleeping impossible. On the nights that are the hardest, I think about Kelly in that crappy vinyl chair, sitting with sand in her ass, legs asleep, and having to pee for the last twelve hours, and I keep going out of respect for what a great mom she is to our kids. I acknowledge the fact that, if our roles were reversed and Kelly was the one staying at home, she would provide daily the same level of care, love, and concern that she did that day. I do what I do because it keeps Arden healthy. I do it because I love her, but I do it the way that I do it with Kelly's example as my guide.

The Saddest That I Have Ever Been

After my father left, when I was thirteen, my baseline for what normal felt like changed. Eventually, I became accustomed to my new normal, and my life seemed to restart. However, until that acclimation happened, my parents' divorce was like a "reality time-out." During that period of my life, I lost the ability to consider everyday things like grades, friends, and the concept of fun. Each day when I woke in the morning, the notion that my parents were divorcing was foremost in my mind, and every step that I took throughout the day reminded me that my father was gone. Every bit of my life was different. We didn't cut the lawn, shop for food, or sit in the house the same way, or at least that's how it seemed. My head always felt like it had been pressurized, my chest felt hollow, and my stomach was in a state of perpetual malaise. I had been impacted so painfully by my parents' divorce that, in the years to come, even the passing of my cherished Gram failed to bring me to such depths. I was sure that nothing could or would ever affect me that way again. Boy, was I wrong.

From the first moment in that summer rental home when Kelly realized that Arden might have type 1 diabetes until, three days later when a nurse tried to teach us how to calculate the amount of insulin Arden would require, I was doing okay. Those days were a furious storm of frantic, with silences so fleeting that there was no opportunity to really think about what was happening. I felt like I was handling the requirements of the situation with at least a bit of aplomb to this point.

Then, the nurse arrived in Arden's room to teach us how to perform the mathematical equations for Arden's meals. The session was going to teach Kelly and me how much insulin was required to keep the food Arden consumes from causing an undesired fluctuation in her blood glucose. The equation was simple, the nurse direct, but

I wasn't grasping it. As soon as Arden left the room and that nurse sat down, I stopped my brain from thinking about anything but what we were about to learn. However, the second that I quieted my mind, fear rushed in. I failed to grasp what the nurse was saying after her first explanation, and before she could try again, I became stupefied by dread, anger, shame, and more pressure to be perfect than I had ever experienced. I wasn't just defeated as I openly sobbed. I felt as though my failure was going to kill Arden.

Kelly was great, and she said all of the right things to help me relax, just like always, but I couldn't focus. Kelly promised the nurse that I wouldn't have a problem picking up what I needed to know and suggested that she could teach me at a better time. The nurse agreed and quietly left Arden's room.

I wish that I could tell you that it only took a few days, weeks, or months to shake the feeling that type 1 diabetes brought to me, but in all honesty, it was much longer. I didn't begin to feel normal again for two years, and the interim was overflowing with new, frightening, and potentially defeating daily situations. Being diagnosed with type 1 diabetes presents an immediate and monumental shift in a caregiver's focus. It doesn't allow for you to get acquainted with your new life. You can't decide to start on Monday, like a diet. If you choose to ignore your new responsibilities, your choice will begin to damage your health immediately. What's worse is that the information you'll require to do a great job of navigating diabetes takes years to accumulate, and the direction that you receive at diagnosis is often less than complete.

One day you're at the beach, and the next someone is telling you that "insulin is the only thing that will keep your daughter alive." As it turns out, insulin is a finicky drug. If you use too much it can end your life, and too little may cause dramatic complications. Those truths create more than a bit of pressure when you use insulin. Try to imagine what it would be like to be told those facts about insulin just before hearing that it will be administered at every meal, snack, and other blood glucose anomaly every day for the rest of your child's life. Really think about that. Every time a person with type 1 diabetes consumes a carbohydrate, he or she must measure, administer, and track an infusion of insulin. That insulin can only be injected under the skin, and each injection is preceded by a blood glucose test that requires a hole to be struck in your finger so that enough blood can be expressed for the test strip to read your blood glucose value.

I once saved every lance and needle that I used for six months of Arden's life with diabetes. More than 1,300 lances were used to create those holes in her fingers, and there were an equal number of needles to go with those tests. I held my two-year-old baby girl and pushed a metal spike into her flesh more than 2,600 times in just those six months. That's more than 5,000 times a year. I did it in the morning when she woke; at breakfast, snack time, and lunch; as a precaution; at dinner; and twice before bed. Due to the fact that type 1 diabetes doesn't rest, I have to slink into Arden's room overnight and test her multiple times as she sleeps.

I don't know if our soul exists in a form that allows a physical description, but mine doesn't look like it did the day before diabetes found us. Each one of those needles—every lance, every drop of blood, every time I measured insulin, every moment of uncertainty and two seizures caused by dosing too much insulin—has dinged my soul. Sometimes the hits aren't too severe, but other times I can feel a piece fall off. Most parents will never know the feeling that comes with the realization that their child may be seconds away from having a seizure because of a decision that they made. Few of us ever have to look at our babies as they rest their heads on their pillows and think as they drift off to dreamland, "Please don't die tonight." Diabetes, a terrible disease that most barely understand, brings you all of that and more. Every moment of every day, every second of every minute, diabetes needs something from you, and if you don't serve it as it requires, it will make you, pay with your life either now or later.

There was a time when I feared losing my son in a store as if that possibility was as real and immediate as any in this world. I now know the difference between those fears and reality. Trust me, there is a significant and omnipresent difference.

Even with that said, my family was not going to live in fear. I wasn't going to live in fear, and there is no way that we were going to allow this shitty hand that we were dealt to take our lives off track for even one second longer than was necessary. People can make claims about how to navigate personal turmoil, and there is a literal ton of books to help you get through life's terrible moments. I only have one piece of advice, and I can lend it to you with the full knowledge that it served me well.

Don't stop and don't give up.

Some days will bring the weight of the world to you—don't stop. There will be times that those days turn into weeks—don't give up. There is a wonderment of understanding on the other side of your struggle, and it's worth getting to. These days and weeks that seem as though they exist only to torture you and the people that you love—they teach. The pain strengthens you and the dings in your soul aren't as deteriorating as they initially seem. In the end, they are reshaping it, and it's up to you to decide what shape it will take.

My mother cried for a week when my dad left us. Then she got up and walked forward. She rarely complained, never looked back, never asked "what if." She took each step into the new unknown with the bravery of a thousand soldiers. Sometimes she cried, yelled, and broke down, but she kept getting back up. She raised my two brothers, Brian and Rob, and me as best she could. We were poor and uncertain from day to day about a great many things, but she never wavered from what she told me as a child. My mom may not have given us all the things that she hoped to, made the money that she desired, or been even the mother that she dreamt of being, but she did a few things perfectly. She kept us together, made sure that we knew that she loved us, and never stopped walking forward, no matter how uncertain her next step was.

I never went to college, and I've had more insanely terrible jobs than you can imagine. I never had a decent car growing up, great clothes, or a new place to live. One could easily make the observation that I grew up without any of the things that a parent should provide, but none of that was what I needed. My mom taught me that families stick together and do the best they can. We are a family and we don't stop. That lesson, perhaps unintended, is my foundation, and it got me through the first two years of Arden's life with type 1 diabetes.

Kelly and I experienced tragedy when Arden was

diagnosed. We learned on the job with diabetes, which led us far too often into disagreements that threatened our relationship. I know that it's tough to disagree with your spouse about parenting complications, education issues, and behavior problems with your children, and we have those issues too. If you take one of those moments and multiply it by a billion, you'll have what it's like to stand in your kitchen at three in the morning with your daughter as her blood glucose plummets.

I remember feeling sure that a glass of milk was the answer to stopping Arden's pending seizure. Kelly believed with all of her heart that the candy in her hand was the only thing that would save our then two-year-old baby from this next potential disaster. We were blind to how fast Arden's blood glucose was falling. As the person who decided to administer the insulin that was causing this low blood glucose incident, I felt horrible. We were all exhausted, in our underwear, and freezing on the cold kitchen tile. Both Kelly and I were riddled with guilt, on edge with parental fear, and positive that we knew best. Live through that and see if you don't plan a visit to the divorce attorney the next morning. Voices became louder, fears heightened, many confusing emotions that didn't seem to belong in the same space with one another were causing conflict.

Suddenly the balloon of terror burst, and we were able to focus completely on Arden. The madness found a lull; we stood in silence holding her and praying that the course we chose would work before the glucose level in her blood dropped far enough that her brain couldn't function. After what seemed like an eternity, the food did its job and the threat passed, but the animosity remained.

These aren't moments that you can talk out. You have to live through them and keep moving forward until you both have enough perspective and context to see them for what they were. It takes a great deal of time to experience and absorb growth such as that. The only thing that will keep you sane, together, and as happy as possible until that time arrives is love. I have daydreamed about throwing Kelly out of a window over the years, and I am one hundred percent sure that she has a hole dug somewhere in our backyard to put me into, but we don't give up. Even when all of our senses say otherwise, and giving up seems like the only option, one of us pushes the other past our dark moment.

Our lives weren't perfect before diabetes, and they certainly aren't now, even though we've found our footing with the disease. I know this may sound strange, but I think diabetes has made us a better family. I say this with deference to all of the possibilities that it has robbed our family of and with thoughtful accounting of the countless adverse health issues that it brings and may bring to Arden. I say that we are stronger now than when we started. I, of course, would trade all of that for Arden to not have diabetes. In fact, I would trade anything, but if she has to live with this burden, at least we've been shown the truth about the resolve and strength that we all have inside. Without diabetes we very well might have lived our entire life without finding out just how much we had to give Cole and Arden.

The saddest I've ever been is my new normal. Barring a medical miracle, Arden will always live with type 1 diabetes. The long-term future of her health will always be uncertain, and the day-to-day fears associated with type 1 will always exist. Kelly and I will never feel like it is permissible to take a break when it comes to thinking about Arden's blood glucose level, and I still cry every once in a while, when all of this becomes too much to bear. There are nights when we don't sleep and days that are consumed with diabetes issues, but they no longer feel sad. Sadness is a state of mind that comes to all of us from time to time. You can choose to stand in it or walk forward and leave it behind. Some sadness, the really persistent type, will follow you as you walk away. But, don't look back. Focus on the good things that you are walking toward and the wonderful people with whom you are walking, because you can be happy anywhere. Remember, where you are at is largely shaped by how you perceive your surroundings and situation.

Learning About Our New Reality

What does any of us really know about the things that we don't live with every day? You can educate yourself as best as you can, but living with something lends the best perspective. One of my lifelong and best friends, Mike, was diagnosed with type 1 diabetes when we were in our late teens, and I never once heard it referred to as juvenile diabetes or type 1 diabetes. Mike just had diabetes. He lived every day with all of the issues that Arden does, but he was relatively private about his condition. Treatments weren't nearly what they are today, so Mike wasn't as frequently involved with his management as we are with Arden's. The most I ever saw of Mike's diabetes was him administering a shot of insulin once or twice a day. Either that was the extent of his care or he was hiding a lot from me.

Mike was my best friend from the time I was sixteen until our lives took on different directions when Kelly and I moved from our hometown. I was with Mike as much as one friend could be with another for the better part of ten years, and still I didn't know very much about diabetes. It's perhaps that fact which makes me tolerant when strangers, extended family members, or friends say the seemingly ignorant and unthinkable things that people sometimes say about type 1 diabetes. When a moment like that happens, I just think back to my years with Mike and remember that I had no idea about type 1 until it came knocking on our front door.

I never opened the book about type 1 diabetes that the hospital gave us. I didn't Google, ask another person, or read a brochure to learn about my daughter's disease. I wish that I could have used those resources, but my mind doesn't work like that. I need to experience the things that I want to learn about firsthand. This made the first two years with type 1 more difficult than perhaps it needed to be. I literally had to experience each moment with type 1 as it came so that I could fully appreciate the inner workings of every issue, treatment, and emergency. My path may have taken longer, but when I emerged on the other side, I was as close to an expert on Arden's physiology and the ways that type 1 affected it as I could hope to be.

There are probably a million people in the world who are better qualified than I am to give a technical explanation of type 1 diabetes, so I would never attempt to do that. I am, however, uniquely qualified to explain how the disease impacts life.

Being told that your child will require an infusion of man-made insulin multiple times throughout the day and night to stay alive is devastating. When you begin to wrap your mind around all of the moments in your day that will require insulin, the feeling intensifies past devastating. It bypasses horrific and settles in at catastrophic. It was explained to us that somehow Arden's body became confused while fighting off a virus and that instead of attacking the virus that she had, her immune system attacked her pancreas. Her pancreas was the organ that made Arden's insulin, but it wasn't going to do that anymore, so we were going to have to provide insulin for her. As much as synthetic insulin is a modern-day miracle and the only reason that my daughter didn't die in a Virginia hospital, it doesn't work exactly like the good stuff that your pancreas makes. Man-made or synthetic insulin takes much longer to begin working and lasts in your body for hours. When I take a bite of an apple, my body senses that intake and releases an amount of insulin that is appropriate for that bite. My insulin acts in my system almost instantaneously and maintains my blood glucose (BG) level. If I didn't have insulin, the bite of apple would begin to drive my BG level up, and it would never come back down. Eventually without insulin I would become very ill, waste away, slip into a coma, and die. What that means is if you could somehow shut your pancreas off right now, the next bite or sip of any substance that contains a carbohydrate would eventually kill you.

Thankfully, synthetic insulin can make your BG level return to normal, but if you take too much, your BG level will fall too low. That state, called hypoglycemia, can rob you of your ability to think clearly and react properly.

Eventually, if left untreated, this low BG level can shut your brain off; you will have a seizure, and without intervention, die. So that's diabetes in a nutshell—too much or too little insulin can end your life.

The variables and situations that seem at times to plot against keeping Arden's blood glucose steady and in range are infinite. I've witnessed her BG level double because she got nervous and fall dangerously fast for reasons that I can't always quantify. Then, there is the problem of food. Most every food has at least a few carbohydrates per serving, and each time something is consumed you have to counter with insulin ... unless you don't. Type 1 is almost impossible to pin down. Arden could eat the same exact food today as she did yesterday, and I could give her exactly the same amount of insulin at the same times, and her BG may react differently than it did the day before.

Good luck figuring out which reaction today will bring. If you consider every time, in the course of a day, that a person ingests a carbohydrate, gets nervous, exercises, or does any number of the hundreds of things that affect your BG level, you'll begin to imagine the enormity of the disease. Even if someone sat down and wrote a book listing every imaginable situation that would affect your BG, the irony of having type 1 is that not every person reacts the same way to these factors, and your diabetes will vary. Diabetes is a twenty-four-hour-a-day moving target.

Arden experiences low BG levels of varying severity almost every day, but the first really severe one whose cause I couldn't decipher happened when she was about three years old. I was thoroughly confused that it had gone so low, as I had followed every protocol as instructed by her endocrinologist. I called the doctor's office later to find out what I had done wrong. I went through the afternoon with the nurse step by step, and neither she nor I could see even a hint of a mistake. After a long silence I said, "So are you telling me that I did everything correct and she still almost had a seizure?" I'll never forget the answer to my question. I say that I'll never forget because it shaped how I think about diabetes. It is a perfect explanation of why the disease is so elusive to the people trying desperately to hold it at bay. The nurse said, "Yeah, that happens sometimes."

I had never heard a more disheartening statement in my life. You may imagine that being told that our child had type 1 diabetes would have been the worst thing that I could hear, but I was without context when the doctors told us that. This was a year later, and now I completely understood what having insulin-dependent diabetes meant. The nurse was telling me that even if I do everything exactly right, once in a while, for reasons that I won't be able to predict, everything may go wrong. I hung up from that call and felt like the world was playing a cruel joke on us.

In the months that followed, we learned more and more lessons each time diabetes decided to teach us one. We survived so many—two seizures, countless low blood glucoses that hovered at the borderline of seizure, high blood glucose values that threatened Arden's long-term health, ignorance, exhaustion, and personal sorrow, to name just a few. A handful of months before the second anniversary of Arden's diagnosis I told myself that we couldn't go on like this much longer. I thought at first that the learning curve would have an end, but if it did, it wasn't in sight.

So, I decided then that if I was going to feel better about diabetes, I would have to respond with more than my "I won't quit" attitude. I had to break myself out of the funk that Arden's diagnosis had drawn us into. What's the saying—"fake it 'til you make it"? I was going to force myself to break free because living in this emotional mess was ripping me apart.

If I had waited to return to our life until I understood every facet of type 1 diabetes, I don't think that I would have ever found my way back. I convinced myself that I had absorbed enough knowledge that I could stop trying to fit life into diabetes and start fitting diabetes into life. So, in the summer of 2008, Arden and I broke out of my self-imposed prison and started to tackle life again. Most moments were uneventful, some were nerve-racking, a few ended as badly as I could imagine, but I'm still here, Arden is still here, and we just keep walking forward.

There was this one warm summer day, Arden and I were out shopping for something, I don't remember what. We were on our way home when I looked back at her in the rearview mirror, and I could instantly tell that something was wrong. Arden looked strange. Her face seemed pliable, she was staring, and so I asked her if she felt okay, but she didn't respond. I realized in an instant that she might be experiencing a low BG level, and I yanked the car onto the shoulder so I could test her blood glucose. I didn't even get out of the car, opting to fling my torso over the seat and test her looking like an overweight circus performer. Her BG was not good, low enough in fact that she wasn't responding like herself. She was combative and angry, which are but a few of the possible signs of hypoglycemia. I began to offer her food and drinks, but she had other ideas. "Ice cream!" she wailed. I tried again to get her to take something that I had on hand, but she was adamant. Every word I spoke just wasted another second that I thought we didn't have. So, I agreed to the ice cream. We were only a few blocks from our house and we had ice cream at home, so I told her that we would go get her some.

"Not that ice cream," she howled, at the top of her lungs. She wanted soft-serve. I didn't think I had a chance at this point to change her mind, so I took off like a mad person across town. We were so close to the ice-cream stand when I was pulled over for speeding, so damn close. I couldn't wait for the officer to saunter up to my window, so I stuck out my hands out where they could be seen, then craned my head out, and began repeating, "My daughter has type 1 diabetes. Her blood sugar is very low, and I'm trying to get her to food ... I have to go." I must have said it three times as he approached. The officer looked into the backseat and saw Arden and her glucose meter. Do you know what he did next? Well, it wasn't give me a police escort to the ice cream stand, that's for sure. He took my license and registration and told me that I could go after he made sure there were no warrants out on me. I was stunned. This was not how it went on C.H.I.P.S. Not only wasn't Arden receiving a lights-and-sirens escort, this guy didn't understand in any way the severity of our situation.

"I have to get out of the car. I need to check her blood sugar again," I told him, as he walked away. I didn't wait for him to answer before I got out. I retested Arden and tried again to talk her into a different snack. Her BG was still falling, and the ice-cream stand was just around the corner. I was equally angry and scared to death. It felt like an eternity until he returned. We made it to the ice-cream stand in time, but that cop sent me a speeding ticket in the mail. This incredibly screwed up moment would have kept me in the house for weeks had it happened the year before, but armed with my new "this is just how it is" attitude, I laughed my way through it ... and I got out of that ticket in court.

The greatest lesson diabetes has taught me is that the struggle makes the living that much more sweet. Living a day with type 1 diabetes demands a level of focus that the average person's day does not. It also puts the need for your active participation in decisions about your health front and center. You can choose to let the disease dictate your life to you, or you can take control by setting your fears aside and leading the way. Before type 1 diabetes, I merely existed through some of the days of my life, happy to let time take me where it would. I might have gone along like that forever if it hadn't been for Arden's diagnosis. I was living life, enjoying my family. I thought I was doing okay, but I never really understood how precious a second was. In the past, it always felt like there was tomorrow, and that feeling, though comfortable, caused me to waste a great deal of time. Now that I understand, not just in theory but also through the eyes of my little girl, how fragile life is, I savor every second like another one isn't coming.

There are a few things in life that defy logic when you measure their impact on you. Marriage, having children, and responsibility are just few, but loving a child with diabetes is the king of putting life into perspective. It isn't often that you can make the legitimate case that something is as wonderful as it is terrible. Maybe the saying "nothing worth having comes easy" would have been a better title for this chapter. I'm in no way saying that I am happy that Arden has this devastating, incurable, chronic illness. All I'm saying is that if something this terrible enters your life and it doesn't kill you, the only way to live well and have the last laugh is to find the good in your situation no matter how deeply it's hidden in the bad.

Writing on the Internet Saved Me

When I was twelve years old, I bought my first computer from RadioShack. I think it was called a TRS-80. The computer didn't have a monitor, so I had to connect it to a television. There was no hard drive, and while there was the ability to save information to an optional cassette recorder, I couldn't afford one. I found a book of program code that you could, wait for it, type in line-by-line to make the computer, you know, do something.

I found this one code in the book that was called something like "exercising man," but don't hold me to that being the exact title for the code. I spent hours typing that code into my TRS-80, and when I was finished and pressed enter all it said was "error." That error message didn't deter me, though. I wanted to be part of the computer revolution so badly that I retyped the code, and this time I stopped every few lines to make sure that I hadn't made a mistake. The exercising man was in reality a stick figure, five lines with a circle over them arranged to look like a man (think hangman). When I finished retyping the code, I pressed enter again and the figure completed one jumping jack—one. Arms up, legs together, and return.

I saved my allowance for that computer for a very long time. To say that that "exercise man" and the experience of getting him to do his one jumping jack was a letdown would be an understatement of epic proportions. I pushed return a few more times, perhaps out of bemusement more than anything else. Then, I shut the computer off, packed it back into its box, and walked it right back to RadioShack. I had deemed this computer "not ready for prime time." The money went back into my drawer and stayed there until the Commodore 64 became available later that year.

I've had a computer every day of my life since that

Commodore, and each advancement in computing has been better than the last. From stick figures that exercise to dot matrix printers, I've loved each step as technology moved forward. My favorite advancement happened for me in the late eighties when I bought a modem. Those who have heard an old modem dial into the Internet will never forget the sound. First you heard the dial tone and then the number dialed, "dee, dee, deet, doot, doot, doot, doot." After a moment of silence, a symphony of electronic sounds, whistles, shrieks, and bells exploded through the tinny speaker. If you were lucky it would connect to the Internet with a string of angry electronic noises. After the connection was made, the modem would go silent, and a timer would begin to run so you knew how long you were online because you were paying for access by the minute. That, my friends, was my first Internet connection, and boy was it slow.

We mainly used the Internet back then for emailing, but there were a few places on the Net to get pictures of things that interested you, although it took almost ten minutes to download one. Today's Internet is a whole lot better for many reasons, but the number-one reason is that there are more people using it. In the beginning, the Internet was amazing just because it existed, and quickly more and more people found email. It became the new way to send a message. Suddenly, we could reach out to people who lived far away without much effort, and the world was about to get smaller.

Even though I'm a visual learner, it still baffles me that Arden's type 1 diabetes diagnosis didn't send me running to my computer to find out more about the disease. Maybe it was a bit of destiny that I didn't go that route, because then I would have found diabetes blogging. Instead of starting my own blog I might have only read someone else's, who knows?

When I began chronicling my life as a type 1 diabetes caregiver in August of 2007, I used a free application called iWeb that came with my Apple computer to post my thoughts on the Internet. The link to the site was long and convoluted, but I didn't care because I was only going to show it to a few close friends and family. My first posts came when I decided that I would write on the site each time that diabetes required me to interact with it for one day. I hoped that if I did so, the people in our lives would better understand how completely diabetes could over-take a life, and that the experience would move them to advocacy.

If you go to my web site today, you can still see the first post that I ever made. It was on August 16, 2007, at three in the morning, seven days before Arden's first diaversary (the anniversary of Arden's diagnosis). Well, someone must have thought my message was worth spreading, because a few weeks later I received an email from a woman in England. She was the mother of a child who also has type 1 diabetes and she wrote to me to lend her support and thank me for being so transparent about our life with type 1.

I didn't know it then, but that woman and I by virtue of my sharing belong to a community online that is affectionately called "The DOC." DOC stands for "Diabetes Online Community," and it's made up of some of the best people whom I've ever met in my life. A virtual community of people with diabetes, parents of children with diabetes, really any person whose life is touched by the disease, whether it be through type 1, type 2, or LADA (Latent Autoimmune Diabetes of Adults). Hell, if you or someone you love has a pancreas that doesn't work, the DOC is the place for you.

The best thing about the DOC is that it isn't a web site, a message board, or a blog. It doesn't exist as a Facebook page or a Twitter handle. It is the metaphysical collection of all of those things combined. When I wrote on the Internet on August 16, my words added themselves to the DOC. Every time someone tweets a link, offers support on a Facebook page, or lends knowledge in a health advocacy chat, that person is participating in and adding to the community.

Not long after I received the email from England, I decided that if what I wrote helped one person, it could perhaps help more, so I purchased the URL www.ardensday.com. I continued to follow the path that I set for myself and wrote about my life as a type 1 caregiver with as much transparency as I could muster. I wrote about everything that happened to us, all of the messy, sad, sometimes wonderful details. The more I wrote, the more people I would hear from. Mostly from parents like us, people who were scared, angry, lost, and in search of answers, advice, and support.

It took me years to really appreciate that "Arden's Day" was as therapeutic for me as it was for the people reading it. I was so focused on helping that I didn't see that I was being helped. The sharing was cathartic, and I was finally writing, which was a lifelong dream. I may have decided that I was coming out of my post-diagnosis fog, but in all honesty, it was that decision in combination with starting my blog that saved me.

A blog is more than a diary even if no one reads it. The act of posting something on the Internet is freeing. It's the physical complement to the idea that saying how you feel out loud can release you from your worry's burden. The greatest surprise that blogging brought to me is the knowledge that when people who are struggling with similar issues read what the writer wrote, they are unburdened as if they had written it themselves. It's the manifestation of the message that you are not alone that makes your shit feel manageable and one of the most amazing things to which I've ever borne witness.

The Internet took my parents' kitchen table and made it available to every person with a computer, tablet, or Internet-ready phone. In the seventies, my parents and their friends would sit around one another's kitchen tables, smoking cigarettes, drinking coffee, and talking for hours on end. Whether you hang out in a bar, go bowling with friends, join a book club, or see a therapist, you are communicating. The act of getting something off of your chest and finding out that you aren't alone, after all, is a basic human need.

The DOC is where I first learned about the brand of insulin that Arden now uses. It's where I found out about continuous glucose monitoring technology and where I gather support when I feel like diabetes is getting the best of me. One night some years ago, I was awake at two in the morning because Arden's blood glucose level was erratic, and I couldn't trust that she'd be okay if I went to sleep. Our house was still and draped in darkness. I would walk into Arden's room every twenty minutes to make sure that her situation was progressing as I hoped. In between my trips, I sat in bed and tried to rest without falling asleep. I didn't have many options to pass time, so at one point I went on Twitter. So many wonderful DOC members use Twitter to communicate, and I planned to pass some time looking at their tweets.

However, before I could start browsing, I saw a mother whom I knew talking about her son's low blood glucose and how she didn't think she was going to get much sleep tonight. I reached out and told her that I was doing the same; we commiserated for a few moments and wished each other luck. I don't know if she was having the same exact experience that I was, but a few tears rolled down my cheek as I shut down the app. I was alone in the dark, exhausted, and tired of diabetes. It may sound trivial, but I hope that it doesn't. The knowledge that another person was doing what I was at that moment and understood how I felt was the inspiration I needed to make it through that night. My tears came when I imagined that my existence in our virtual world might have meant the same to her.

I have been fortunate enough to meet some of these people in real life, and I have to say that not one of them has been less than amazing, all in their own way and somehow together as one. The DOC has been around for much longer than I've been a part of it, and it grows every day—it is a place where you can seek friendship, support, and answers just as easily as you can provide them. Its existence helps countless people in endless ways. I am but a very small part of the DOC, and yet when I think about its value in the world, I feel the pride of a thousand proud fathers.

Communication, sharing, chatting with a friend, it doesn't matter what you call it, or what vehicle you use to accomplish it—just do it. Tell someone what burdens you, and it will cease being a problem. It's only with the clarity that an unburdened mind has to offer that you will be able to extract as much joy from life as you deserve, and I think you deserve as much as your heart can hold.

His
Last Chapter

If you are reading this and did not skip ahead, or are not in any way related to me, please accept my sincere thanks!

The process of writing has allowed me the pleasure of thoughtfully reliving the moments in my life that I considered poignant when they occurred. That indulgence felt like someone granted me a time-out from life and then showed me home movies of every impactful moment through which I ever lived. I wasn't able to speak about them all with you, but I want to thank you for reading the ones that fit in this book. I've tried to relay them to you in a way that reflects the simple but hidden truths about raising a family while living well. I hope you have time for just one more story …

I was estranged from my father for most of my life and only reconnected with him in his last few years because of a kind woman whom he met named Martha. Martha made my dad reach out to his sons, and though our wounds never fully healed, her actions allowed me to be at his side when he passed away. Writing this book gave me the time and inclination to remember my life in detail. That process allowed me to thoughtfully relive the lessons that each of my days has taught me.

There were four people in the hospital room for my father's last few hours on this Earth. Martha, myself, the son of the woman he left my mother for, and that man's wife. The other people present seemed to love my father as I remember loving him when I was a child. They looked at him in the way that I was never able to re-create after he left us. It made me sad for a few moments, but then I felt happy for him. I was glad that he felt love in his life, even after his presence left mine. I expected to be angry when I recognized that these people had the connection with my father that I longed for, but I just wasn't. It was too late for that now. I can't take credit for my response. I didn't have it purposely, but I am grateful for it as it shaped how I experienced the next five hours.

My father called me to his bedside around two in the morning. He took my hand and told me, "I think I'm doing the right thing." I didn't know what he meant, but I answered that I thought he was, too. I told him, "Dad, you should do whatever makes sense for you. I think you are doing the right thing, too." Then he reached for the call button with his other hand, never letting go of mine.

It took a few minutes for the nurse to arrive, and I tried to live an entire lifetime in those minutes. My father was squeezing my hand the way I remembered him doing when I was a little boy. We never spoke; I just looked at his face and tried to remember every happy moment with him from my childhood that I could, because I feared that I knew why he pushed that button. When the nurse arrived, he told her it was time, that he couldn't take the pain. She simply said okay and smiled at my dad, with a sadness that I remembered from another nurse's face. She looked at him the same way the nurse who retrieved us from the waiting room on the day of Arden's diagnosis with type 1 diabetes did. I held his hand until the medication made him fall asleep, and then I sat in a chair and made awkward small talk with the people whom he found after he left us. He died peacefully just before sunrise.

The others left a few minutes after he passed, but I stayed behind in the room with my father because I couldn't make my legs move. I felt like I was thirteen again, and I wanted to sit on our sofa with our family portrait just a little longer.

I stood quietly at first and cried, but when I eventually stopped crying, I didn't leave as I had thought I would. Instead, I began to talk to him and tell him a few of the stories about my life that I wished he had known. I told him the stories that I thought would make him happy to know. I told him the ones that I thought would have made him come home if he had only known them all of those years ago. I talked about Kelly and our kids. I explained how much I missed him growing up, and that I would look out the window at night hoping that he would come home. I put my hand on his foot before I told him that I was a good dad to my children, and that I thought that his leaving was why I try so hard. I thanked him for that, and then I told him that I loved him and that I was sorry that I was leaving him alone.

It took me five more minutes before I could stop looking at his face and make my legs carry me from that room. I stood for those minutes in silence as tears streamed from my eyes. I wasn't really crying anymore, but they just wouldn't stop flowing. I finally felt that if I didn't leave, I never would. So I broke that silence by saying, "I love you." I closed my eyes really tight and tried to imagine one more time the moments in my life that he missed as if I thought I could transfer them through the sheet so he could take them with him. "I love you, Dad ... I wish you were there." And with that, I let go of his foot and slowly began walking out of the room. I stopped in the doorway and looked back at him one last time.

My poor father was lying dead in a hospital bed. My mom wasn't there, his other sons weren't there, no one that he was related to by blood or marriage was in attendance at his death. The only person who stayed with him was his adopted son. A person that he took as his own when he was only a baby. He told me I was wanted, and then spent thirteen years making me believe it was true. Then he spent the rest of his life doing the opposite. I wondered what he thought about while he held my hand before the nurse came into the room. Did he know that he repaired our relationship with just his touch?

He made so many mistakes in the years after he began his family, but only one of them ended up actually hurting us—he gave up. The minute that he decided to come back, we were a family again. For a few hours on the morning of my father's death, I sat in a room with three people who had been unjustly given my life. Still, I was as happy as I'd ever been as I sat with them and waited for my dad to die. For a few hours that day, I had a father who loved me and I knew it. That's the message I tried in vain to tell to my dead father before I left that room, and it's the same message that I am trying to impart to you.

When I arrived home it was still early in the morning and no one was awake yet in our house. I looked in on the kids and then I climbed back into bed, my eyes burning from no sleep and too many tears. I felt weak and exhausted. I moved my body slowly trying not to wake Kelly, but once I was settled, I couldn't stop myself from taking her hand. Her skin felt heavenly, and her touch relieved my anguish. As my hand covered Kelly's I thought, "Our life isn't perfect but we could make it."

I felt like we had to, that we should, that I wanted to. I don't know what the meaning of life is—maybe it's far too complex to put into words. I think that our day-to-day minutiae cloud why we are all here. I know that it's too easy to lose sight of what's important. There are days when I do or say things that defy logic. It's inevitable that we'll make mistakes and that time will pull us from where we mean to be. There really is only one thing you can do to stop these forces from changing your destiny—don't give up.

Life tries so hard to show us that everything is possible, but so often we give up anyway. All any family needs is one person to say "I'm not giving up." It only takes one person to break a cycle and refuse to stop moving forward, but it requires a lifetime of commitment to see that goal through. My father couldn't do it, his father couldn't do it, but I'm going to. I'm going to be the dad that my dad wanted and didn't get. I'm going to be the dad he started out being, but couldn't sustain.

Why me? Why don't I just kick that can a little farther down the road and let Cole deal with it? I've thought a lot about that question. I don't love my family more than my dad did. I'm not a better person than he was. It's not intelligence, money, or education that showed me the light. Simply, I opened my heart. I let myself feel. I listen, even though Kelly doesn't think I do sometimes, as she tries to teach me what our family needs. The rest came from my children. Seeing them born and then understanding that I was going to be responsible for not just keeping them alive, but guiding them to who they will one day become, fuel me. There were plenty of moments when I could have given up and times when I actually considered it.

Before my father passed away, I didn't give up because I never wanted my children to feel the piercing, numbing, unrelenting sadness that accompanies the dissolution of a family. That reason will live with me always, but since his death I know there is more to it. Kelly and I have a connection with our children and each other that only comes from being a family. It's incredibly regrettable that my father and I didn't learn until the very end that our connection could repair any bridge that he destroyed in our past, but now I know. I don't give up because nothing is as bad as giving up. I may have learned that tough lesson the day that my dad died, but I was able to absorb, understand, and retain it because I'm a stay-at-home dad. I learned to see the world the way mothers do. Open your heart, and your family will fill it with a glorious feeling that transcends description.

Acknowledgments

Lynne Johnson, we ended up on the phone together through happenstance, and that meeting made one of my dreams a reality. Thank you for shepherding me through the process of writing in book form. Your guidance and vision were gifts that I'll always hold dear. I can't imagine a better publishing partner.

Jeremy Sterling, thank you for being my sounding board when I doubted myself, got overly excited, or just needed to hear myself talk. You should have charged a co-pay.

Spry Publishing, for the opportunity of my lifetime, thank you.

I've been fortunate to spend time with a few amazing

storytellers. I want them to know that I learned how to hold a room's attention by listening to their cadence and watching their body language, faces, and eyes as they captured audiences. I could never tell a joke like "Uncle" Frank. You were masterful, sir, and I miss watching you weave. Bob Lewis, your stories had so much energy, and you told them with the most intense pleasure. Hand gestures, sound effects, I felt your joy. To my middle school English teacher, David Joffe—I never took your class seriously, and for that I am both sorry and regretful. I was, however, always captured by your confidence. You commanded the floor, were unapologetic in your seriousness, and sarcastic in a way that I still hold dear. I never read the books you asked me to, but know this: I felt terrible about not doing so.

The ability to say how you feel in a way to which others are drawn and pay attention is an art form. Finding a way to deliver your message so that it adds itself to the consciousness of your audience—now that is a superpower. I've been forever impacted by the thoughts, feelings, and beliefs of a few people who exist for me as entertainers, authors, and musicians, but they are so much more. They are Howard Stern, Kevin Smith, Yo-Yo Ma, Eminem, Malcolm Gladwell, David Foster Wallace, and Dr. John Sarno.

Howard Stern, his radio show, and the talented people who work on it taught me how to speak in an interesting way. Stern showed me that boundaries should be pushed, that norms should be challenged, and, most of all, that everyone has a story and that each one is incredibly detailed, interesting, and worth hearing. Howard, Robin, Fred, Gary, Jackie, Artie, and everyone else who has ever worked on *The Howard Stern Show*, thank you so very much for all of the years. What a pleasure, what a lesson. I'm not sure where I'd be without your voices in my life.

I first met Kevin Smith when he asked on his web site for fans to attend the filming of DVD extras for his movie *Mallrats*. Kevin let me watch for hours as they filmed interview after interview. It was in that room that I realized he and I weren't all that different. It was the moment when I started believing that people like me could do something special. Kevin, and I mean this in the best way, that was my *Slackers* moment. I would never have dared to dream of writing without your influence. Thank you for being so accessible, so real, and so transparent with your feelings. Generations of fans owe you more than this thank-you can express.

Thank you to Yo-Yo Ma and Eminem for letting your souls out through music. You both add a catharsis to the world that is, for me, unmatched. Both soothe my soul in very different ways. Yo-Yo Ma, when you play the cello, it draws out every emotion I have. With your guidance the strings on your cello make me smile, think, cry, and feel. I'm not exactly sure what I feel when you play, but the sensations transcend explanation. They defy words. I know this for sure. My life would not be as rich without those feelings, and it's your cello that brings them to me. You are a gift.

Eminem's words, phrasing, and emotions move me. His willingness to let us see into his mind's eye captures me, I'm thankful for it. He is a modern-day poet, and his music is as impactful to me as Ma's cello. Though his life's struggles are different than mine, I closely identify with the pain that he feels as he tries to understand them.

Mike McKeon, your presence in my life is, was, and

forever will be monumental. I love you like a brother.

I have so many beautiful friends who have impacted me. I can't name you all, but please know that each of you has made an indelible mark on my soul. You've shaped who I am and guided me with your friendship. My life would not be the same without each of you in it.

Thank you to the diabetes online community for being there.

My mother Beverly and my brothers Brian and Rob: our memories are my foundation. I hope that you will always know how much I love you. Brian, I never should have made you walk home to change the channel. Rob, I'm sorry both for tossing you into our front yard naked and for giving you that Bruce Lee–themed nickname. You guys are the best brothers in the world. Mom, thank you for never giving up. You're a rock, a fantastic mother, and a light in all of our lives.

Cole, your arrival signaled the start of my life as it was meant to be. Each day with you brings me more joy than I could have ever imagined possible. I love you. Your smile lightens my heart, and the sound of your voice brings meaning to my days. I am forever proud of all that you are, feel, and think. Thank you for being my son. This book, my life, really everything wouldn't be as wonderful without you. I can't wait to see the man you will become.

Arden, by showing me your strength, I found mine. You move through life with a beauty and grace that transcends your age and experience. I love you with all that I am. Your playful attitude, sharp wit, and perfect face bring me to a new level of what a father's heart can feel and hold each day. I'm excited to see the woman you will one day be. You are the smartest, bravest girl, and I'm so very proud of you. Thank you for touching me so deeply in my heart.

Kelly, I never thought that a girl like you would fall for my bullshit. Thanks for taking a chance. We really made something great together. You're my best friend, and your gaze still stops me in my tracks. I can only imagine how much I must bug the crap out of you after all of these years ... but you're a good sport, and I appreciate that you haven't smothered me with a pillow. You were the first person to believe me when I said I wanted to write, and you never lost that belief even when you were long past thinking that I ever would. Thank you for being the best girlfriend, wife, mother, and friend that a guy could ask for. Thank you for our family, for the kids, for our life. Your dedication to our family and persistence throughout our life is staggering. I'll never be able to repay you for all that you've given me, but I promise to die trying. I love you with all my heart.

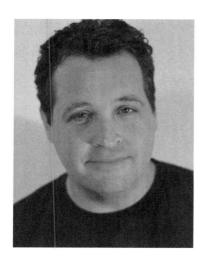

Scott Benner is a stay-at-home father, a diabetes advocate, and a keen observer of the human condition. He has spent the last twelve years raising his two children at their family home in New Jersey.

Scott shares his triumphs and challenges in parenting a child with type 1 diabetes on ArdensDay.com, an inspirational blog for parents and caregivers of children with diabetes. His first book, Life Is Short, Laundry Is Eternal, is a perfect blend of Scott's passion for parenting, his knack for positivity in the face of adversity, and his exceptional skill at spinning a yarn.

Scott finds wisdom, love, and a deeper understanding of life by paying close attention to the pauses in between the moments that make up our lives. He enjoys those pauses—and the busy times that intervene—with his wife Kelly, son Cole, and daughter Arden.

Blogs

www.scottbenner.com

www.ardensday.com

Facebook

www.facebook.com/LifeIsShortLaundryIsEternal

www.facebook.com/ArdensDay

Charity

www.ardensdaygives.org

Twitter

@ArdensDay